Why is it so difficult to die?

This book is dedicated to my mother Robina, who taught me so much about people; my father Sylvester who is lying in his death bed at the age of 90 as I finish writing this book; my wife Priscilla for being my love and support over the past 20 years and my children, Pamela and Neville for making me smile each day I live

Why is it so difficult to die?

Brian Nyatanga

Quay
Books

Mark Allen
Publishing Ltd

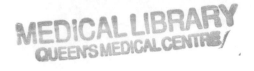
Quay Books Division, Mark Allen Publishing Ltd
Jesses Farm, Snow Hill, Dinton, Wiltshire, SP3 5HN

British Library Cataloguing-in-Publication Data
A catalogue record is available for this book

© Mark Allen Publishing Ltd 2001
ISBN 1 85642 046 9

Printed in the UK by The Cromwell Press, Trowbridge, Wiltshire

Contents

Contributors

Jean Bayliss MA (Counselling), BG Dip (Counselling in educational settings), ALAM

After a background in education she was head of department in a further education college. At present she works as a counsellor and trainer, with a special interest in loss and grief. She is currently promoting clinical supervision to support practitioners in hospices, hospitals and trusts.

Simon Chippendale M Med Sci (Health Care Ethics), BSc (Hons), RGN, RNT, Cert Ed, Dip Pall Nursing

Simon Chippendale completed his Masters in Medical Science in 1996 at the University of Birmingham. Prior to his current post at his local hospice he worked within palliative care education with a national cancer charity and at the University of Birmingham. He is committed to providing palliative education that influences practice and to developing understanding of ethical issues.

Craig Gannon MB, ChB, MRCGP, Dip Pall Med

Having completed his medical training in Birmingham he worked as a general practitioner before completing specialist training in palliative medicine. He is now a part-time consultant.

Brian Nyatanga MSc, PG Dip, Cert Ed, DIPSN, Dip Psychology, ENB 931, RGN

Brian Nyatanga is a Macmillan Senior Lecturer at the University of Central England, Birmingham. He has ten years of clinical and educational experience in palliative care and has written extensively on this area for the nursing press.

Acknowledgements

It is always dangerous ground to try and acknowledge everyone by name, as a name is often unintentionally omitted. Firstly, in a general way, I would like to thank everyone who has helped me with this book, whether it was directly or indirectly. A special mention must go to all the contributors; Dr Craig Gannon, a dear friend and colleague of seven years, Simon Chippendale my successor at St Richard's Hospice, Worcester where I started the ideas for this book and Jean Bayliss, my previous clinical supervisor, mentor and professional friend. I owe a lot to Jean's belief in me and all her support during difficult times and mind mapping exercises.

I would also like to thank; Celia Robinson for her help with the case study in *Chapter 6,* Karamat Hussain and Mr S Aujla for their help when I was writing *Chapter 7,* and Hilary Al Rasheed for the cost details of funerals in *Chapter 8.* I am grateful for the exchange of experiences of dying and death through my discussions with Taro Takeshima and Haruo Obara from Japan. This certainly gave me another dimension to think about.

My thanks to Rachel Bucknall for believing in me and giving me my first opportunity in palliative education, Dr Richard Woof for his challenging ideas, and Professors David Field and David Cox for helping to formulate the initial ideas for this book.

Without the typing skills of my former and present secretaries, Lynne Neel and Jane Trinham respectively this book would not have been finished. A great many drafts were typed out for proof reading. I am grateful also to my critical friend, Steve Challinor, now in Singapore, for proof reading the drafts.

My last acknowledgement is for my educational mentor and friend, Debbie Spencer, for her guidance in my early days in palliative care education. And finally, I would like to thank all the patients and their families who shared their experiences, stories (often painful ones) with me during my clinical work, from which I gained so much knowledge. I am even more grateful now that I am able to share this knowledge with others.

Brian Nyatanga
June, 2000

Foreword

Brian Nyatanga and his colleagues are to be congratulated on the comprehensiveness and timeliness of this excellent text. How we support our dying clients and, indeed, how we accomplish the process of dying either for our loved ones or even for ourselves is a universal concern.

Nuland (1993) notes that,

The greatest dignity to be found in death is the dignity of the life that preceded it.

(p. 243)

By its sound integration of practice and theory, this book makes a major contribution to promoting an enhanced understanding of how to maintain dignity. As human beings we should be interested in and concerned about the way that the act of dying is achieved. There are many factors that can make dying so difficult for all concerned. This book discusses these factors openly and sensitively, and helps the reader (carer) appreciate the psychosocial, spiritual and ethical issues involved in death and dying. I would recommend this book to everyone who shares these views and concerns and wishes to further, not only their knowledge but also their compassion so that in the end we all do better.

Roswyn Hakesley-Brown
Author and consultant in healthcare education

Reference

Nuland SB (1993) *How we die*. Chatto and Windus, London

Introduction

Although death is the only certainty in life, people have different perceptions and different attitudes towards death and dying. Death has been seen (particularly in the western world) as a taboo topic, although there are suggestions that this is no longer the case. If this is so, then the absence of this taboo should be more evident in palliative care settings where death tends to occur more often than in other settings. However, from my clinical experience working in palliative care, the evidence points to the fact that death is still not always talked about openly by the dying person and his/her family. On the other hand, it is accurate to suggest that the advent of palliative care itself has led to an increase in discussing death, but this is more so of healthcare professionals working within this setting.

A taboo, for purposes of clarification and in the case of death, is something that is too horrible to even talk or think about. There is a simplistic view which believes that by not talking about death it will somehow be averted. There is something about death that makes it both difficult to talk about and to deal with the emotions it provokes.

This book attempts to offer a possible rationale and discussion on why dying (as a process that leads to death) is difficult to negotiate. It argues using philosophical and psychological perspectives and shows why it is difficult for people to die, hence the title. More ground has already been covered in American literature on this topic, but we need to understand it from our own perspective, therefore the focus of the book is British. A sensitive but honest approach to death and dying is taken, as death can be a painful experience for most people. The book also aims to persuade readers to understand themselves first in the face of death, examining their own attitudes and beliefs, and then perhaps begin to view death and its inevitability in a different way.

The way a dying person may wish to negotiate his/her own passage from this life is explored, helping the healthcare professional to understand this person more fully and hopefully provide better quality care. *Chapter 6* offers practical information and suggestions on how to care for a dying person and his/her family, establishing a balance between understanding the philosophical and psychological perspective of dying and what can be done in practice to help the dying person achieve a personal, dignified death.

Palliative care is defined by the World Health Organization (1990) as:

> *The total care of patients whose disease is no longer responsive to curative treatment and in which the control of pain, of other symptoms, and of the psychological, social and spiritual problems are paramount.*

The goal being the best quality of life for patients and their families. Such care provision is most effective when carried out by a well co-ordinated multi-professional team. The different levels of palliative care (generalist palliative care and specialist palliative care) provision are discussed briefly in *Chapter 3*.

Healthcare professional students and those undertaking continuing education programmes in palliative care, as well as practitioners working in a variety of settings where death occurs, will find this book a useful aid. The Office of National Statistics identified these settings and published its figures in 1997. The percentages of places where death occurred in England and Wales were identified as; NHS Hospitals 53.3%, private nursing homes 24.2%, hospices 3.4%, and psychiatric hospitals 0.8%. It was found that 10% of deaths occurred in non-NHS hospitals with a further 8.4% dying in other establishments including patients' own homes. These figures show how death occurs in almost every setting, making this book useful reading for practitioners working in these areas.

It is important for the reader to appreciate the theoretical underpinnings of this book, but without losing sight of the uniqueness of the individual who is dying.

Setting the scene

The first chapter is a brief overview of attitudes and their formation in general. This is followed by a close scrutiny on attitudes towards death between the twelfth and twentieth centuries. This will help to understand the transformation that has taken place in such attitudes over time. This transformation is an indication of peoples' awareness of themselves and their degree of individuality.

Chapter 2 discusses the notion of a paradigm of death, and whether there is one. This leads on to an exploration of a death system and the factors that shape it, including an in depth discussion on the philosophical and psychosocial and spiritual definitions of death. Examples are used to explain complex philosophical arguments which helps to elucidate information and aid understanding while remaining reader friendly. This chapter also argues that a death fear is common in our society, explaining its origin. A detailed discussion of the contexts of awareness based on the thinking of Glaser and Strauss explains this paradigm of death.

The following chapters, (*3 and 4*) focus on the perceived medicalisation of dying. Dr Gannon, a consultant in palliative medicine, argues the ethical position taken by medicine in caring for patients. It is usually difficult to be critical of your own profession publicly, but a finely balanced and objective view of the role of palliative medicine in the care it provides to the dying patient and family is given.

If we are not careful as professional carers, there is a tendency to make the patient dependent on us (for the wrong reasons) for all their needs. A pragmatic approach would be to enable the patient to be self-reliant and to gain as much independence as his/her illness allows. It may be quite comforting to be needed by the patients we care for as long as what we do does not stop a patient regaining some of the lost control and independence caused by illness.

Chapter 5 examines the ethical issues surrounding dying and death, and offers a starting point for the principles of health ethics. The discussion centres on the issue of sanctity versus quality of life. This chapter also looks at dying ethically, thereby highlighting the dilemmas faced by the dying patient, carers and professionals.

Having considered the difficult issue of ethical dying, *Chapter 6* offers the reader practical ways of caring for the dying patient, showing different ways that the patient may go through his/her dying using the PEPSSI approach. A few examples are given to help the reader to try and work out how best to help the patient and his/her family.

Chapter 7 offers an extra dimension in caring for the dying patient by exploring some cultural variations encountered by carers and professionals in dying and death. This chapter utilises the fact files already established for each cultural group. Use of such fact files should not be taken as endorsement of the inherent stereotypical assumptions, but only as a way of offering a starting point for discussion on the topic. This chapter argues that there has been a kaleiodoscope of cultures and therefore it is unfortunate to hold stereotypical views about the original culture, for example Muslim or Jewish. The argument centres on the pluralist society that we live in,where cultures are bound to change either through acculturation or enculturation. What is more important in this chapter is the consideration of what happens during dying and death even for those cultures that have undergone acculturation. The chapter ends by offering suggestions on how to care for patients from different cultures.

Chapter 8 discusses the role of funerals and tries to answer the question, 'Are funerals and their rituals functional or dysfunctional for the bereaved?' The idea of living with the dead is explored, showing how the dead may still keep a hold on the living. The role of obituaries is examined as is that of funeral directors, again highlighting how dying and death has become a business of others. This leads on to support the claim of the book that it is difficult to die in today's society.

The final chapter discusses why it is important to think about loss and grief. Jean Bayliss looks at the staged theories and models of helping the bereaved cope with their grief. The shortcomings of these theories and models are highlighted, and alternative ways of helping the bereaved are proposed, moving away from focusing on grief as being pathological, to being something that people can and should grow around. This chapter introduces new models and draws from research work carried out in New Zealand, The Netherlands and the United Kingdom on helping the bereaved come to terms with their loss at their own pace. The chapter offers a succinct summary of post-death activities. At the end the reader is left with new ideas, but for inflexible practitioners, this chapter may be a real challenge. There is a need to move away from working with order (staged theories and models) and allow chaos to prevail so that the bereaved can find their own order.

All the contributors and myself genuinely believe that this book is both informative and sensitive in discussing such a complex topic. The final goal is to share ideas (or in the words of my Eastern European colleagues, allow for 'sensibilisation') for the benefit of the dying patient and family. If we can help to eradicate or minimise those aspects that make dying so difficult it would be a great legacy to leave behind in palliative care.

Brian Nyatanga
June, 2000

1

Attitudes towards death and dying

Brian Nyatanga

When a person is born we rejoice, and when they are married, we jubilate, but when they die, we pretend that nothing happened.

Margaret Mead, 1949

The term attitude seems to be used loosely and in different settings so much that its meaning has become rather vague, as will be demonstrated in this chapter. It seems a logical starting point that before exploring attitudes towards death, it may be worthwhile clarifying this term — attitude. You have probably heard people making comments such as, 'I don't like his attitude', 'He has got an attitude problem' or 'They will not tolerate that kind of attitude in this community'. We read about the attitude of western countries towards certain issues like abortion, human rights and more recently fox hunting as barbaric. We have also heard about some people in the developing countries who, apparently, have no attitude at all towards most of the above mentioned issues. When used in these different ways the term attitude lacks a universal meaning. However what seems to be universal in all the above examples is the reference made to viewpoints of either individuals or communities. Where a community is involved, this may refer to a collective viewpoint of that group of people. If we use the individual viewpoint, it can be seen that by not liking somebody else's attitude, this may suggest that he or she is not conforming to the expected norm. We should also consider that in such circumstances, perhaps the problem lies with how a person interacts with another person's behaviour.

Defining attitudes

The literature suggests that there is not one definition for 'attitude'. However from all the definitions including a sample given below, common elements emerge that would be useful to our understanding of attitudes. The first element is the way in which an individual believes and thinks about something, in this case it may be death or an activity such as fox hunting. This mental or thought process is the cognitive dimension of an attitude. The second element is the affective dimension, which is how an individual feels about an issue or an object. In this case feelings are to do with how favourable or unfavourable someone or something is to the individual.

The final and common element is how the individual will respond or overtly react, the behavioural dimension, towards the situation or object. Secord and Backman (1964) claim that the behavioural component is based on both cognitive and affective elements. It is now generally accepted that attitudes help us to predict possible behaviour (Fishbein and Ajzen, 1980) although not that accurately.

Sample of definitions

> *An attitude is a mental and neural state of readiness, organised through experience, exerting a directive or dynamic influence upon the individual's responses to all objects and situations with which it is related.*
>
> (Allport, 1935)

> *An attitude is a predisposition to act in a certain way towards some aspect of one's environment, including other people.*
>
> (Mednick *et al*, 1970)

> *Attitudes are likes and dislikes.*
>
> (Bem, 1979)

Beliefs, values and attitude

Using the affective dimension of attitude, it can be seen that this is made up of values and beliefs held by an individual. In this blend, beliefs would represent the knowledge a person has about a situation, in this case death, regardless of the actual accuracy or completeness of that knowledge. Such a belief may influence a person to link things to some attribute. For example, it is well known that Paris is linked with romance, hence Paris is seen as a romantic city, London as money, and death is often equated with suffering and pain.

From a belief follows a value, that is what a person views as desirable and worthwhile. Here there is an element of preference, which becomes a precursor to action. It follows therefore that values, unlike beliefs, which are non-evaluative and neutral, help a person to set standards to guide actions in order to achieve those values. According to Elms (1976) a combination of these two elements (beliefs and values) result in attitude. What must be clear at this point is that all these elements, including affective and cognitive aspects, are factually hypothetical constructs as they cannot be observed or measured accurately, only inferred from the observed behaviour or from listening to the other person's accounts/narratives. Behaviour itself is something that is learned through interacting with immediate family, peers, institutions and the social network. Morgan (1995) makes the point that a person is socialised into an attitude by his/her culture. However, the attitude would remain intact and in its purist form provided that the original culture is not exposed to other cultures. Exposure would result in modification of the original culture (Nyatanga, 1997), a process referred to by DeVito (1992) as acculturation.

Development of attitudes

The understanding of attitudes is an important part of social psychology, perhaps because they (attitudes) are formed and influenced by families, social groups and institutions. This topic is vast and cannot be covered adequately here, only a brief overview is intended. Attitudes develop from childhood experiences through to adulthood and can effect a person's relationship with another. Children often have a naive and simplistic approach to the unknown such as death. In most cases children experience their first death through the 'loss' of an animal (family pet). The way such a death is handled depends mainly on parental influences, as parents tend to shape children's attitudes. Most children tend to use their parents as points of reference. Morgan *et al* (1979) give an example, 'Mama tells me not to play with white boys' or 'Daddy says black people are lazy' (p.453). In this case, Morgan argues that there is a sizeable correlation between children and their parents' attitudes, although specific to religion and politics.

While parental influence subsides as children grow older, social influences become more evident in adolescence. Between the age of twelve and thirty, most attitudes stabilise, in other words they are formed. Sears (1969) called this the critical period. This is also referred to as crystallisation, which commonly applies closely to adults: the shaping of attitudes affecting specifically the adolescence stage. An adolescent's attitude may vary as it is not yet strongly held. As young adulthood approaches (ie. moving into the twenties) most young people begin to make commitments. They may decide to vote in general elections, finish their education and start specialising in a particular career, and others choose to get married. These commitments are made on the basis of the attitudes they hold, which tend to be crystallised and may not change much afterwards.

Crystallisation of attitudes tends to create a need for consistency between attitudes and other information received. It is common to find people changing their attitudes in order to reduce any apparent discrepancy or disharmony. For example, any information that is not consistent within attitudes may demand two possible reactions so as to reduce the disharmony created:

- explaining away (rationalise) that information and demonstrating intrinsically that it is not creating any dissonance
- modifying or changing original attitudes to make them more favourable to the new information, thus reducing such dissonance.

Attitudes are also affected by peers, ie. those of the same age range and educational level. Peers strongly influence the development of attitudes during adolescence, when less time is spent with parents, hence this 'see-saw effect'. Peers are powerful influences and adolescents see them as authorities, people they like to be around, doing things that are 'fun' and different from parental teaching.

Education, information and attitude development

Education tends to play a major part in attitude formation, although this also depends on how far one is educated. There is evidence to suggest that people with more education hold liberals views (Sears, 1969) and are very often of a high socio-economic status. The argument may be whether such liberal views make such people more accepting of their own death or not. They seem to be open-minded with most things in life but death poses a different challenge of immediate non-existence.

Information through exposure to television also contributes to attitude formation. In modern societies, television is the main influential medium in two main ways:

• it plays a considerable part in weakening parental influence
• it portrays images and events vividly and explicitly to adolescents. Today, young people are more aware of what is happening around the world than they were a decade ago.

Attitudes to religion and death

Religion is thought to play a significant part in relieving the fear of impending death (Malinowski, 1965). Indeed, the relief of such fear by religion can be applied to any crisis situation or experience. Malinowski claims that the function of religion is to bring about a restoration of normality to the person experiencing the crisis. The question is what happens to those who do not believe in any religion (eg. agnostics who differ from atheists in that they feel that the concept of a God existing is too abstract to even discuss; their stance on the subject is silence).

But first we need to explore how religion can provide individuals with a means of dealing with crisis situations or phenomena. It is plausible to suggest that death itself is the phenomena that calls for a religious intervention. At the same time death is seen and accepted as the punishment for the sin committed by Adam and Eve in the Garden of Eden. Following after Adam and Eve, the individual is now born into sin and arguably is spiritually flawed. The religious individual may find that religion provides him with more meaning and purpose in the last days of his life. For the religious, death may be seen as providing the passage (pre-determined by a higher power) to eternity. The belief in a God or Higher Power becomes the influencing factor in providing equanimity for the dying person and his family.

There are other contrary views to this sacerdotal perspective, for example Radcliffe-Brown (1965) claims that religion actually causes more anxiety in the dying person because of worrying about God's judgement, the possibility of going to hell and whether his/her life was lived according to the expectations of the religion or ritual. There are two points to make from Radcliffe-Brown's perspective. Firstly, the conclusion that being religious could lead to dysfunctional consequences when faced with death; and secondly, that the non-religious or less religious individual would experience less fear or anxiety about his/her own death. Both Malinowski and Radcliffe-Brown make valid points, but these should not be taken simplistically. Malinowski's theory focuses on the individual's perception of how religion functions for him, whereas Radcliffe-Brown bases his on society, in that society itself expects the dying person to be anxious and fearful of his own death. When viewed like this, it can be argued that religion has an influence on ways of social integration. If it (religion) works for the individual, then it is also working for society.

On the other hand, and if you subscribe to Radcliffe-Brown's perspective, the claim is that religion is a catalyst that creates a sense of anxiety or fear, but this is positive because it helps to maintain the social structure of society.

Let's turn briefly to those who do not believe in God or a Higher Power, because they too negotiate their own dying. People like agnostics have a belief that we probably do not fully understand and they utilise this in the face of death.

Their meanings of death together with those of religious people tend to be socially ascribed. Death in itself is neither fearful nor non-fearful.

It is also true to suggest that in some cases the religious person may find the threat of death so immense that he may be 'forced' to forsake his beliefs for something that is the very opposite of his original beliefs. It is also plausible to suggest that the meanings ascribed to death in any given religion or culture are transmitted to individuals in the society through socialisation.

Death attitude

Having discussed general attitude, we should now focus the discussion on death attitude. This attitude is three dimensional, that is, cognitive, affective and behavioural and therefore helps to present a complete picture of how the individual would deal with aspects and questions relating to death, dying, bereavement and notions such as euthanasia.

Attitudes may involve feelings about dependency, pain, dignity, isolation, rejection, parting from loved ones, after-life and facing the unknown (Morgan, 1995). These feelings and reactions tend to be expressed in different ways, by different people and at different times. Some people may talk very openly about their own death to the extent of making post-death arrangements, while others may avoid talking about it as if silence about death will prevent it from happening. Another way of explaining this death avoidance is to look at the different attitudes as a reflection of the different conceptions of what it is to be a person. This notion of existentialism also forms the basis of spirituality and the relationship of the person to his or her community, the world, to God or a Higher Power. This concept of being a person will be discussed in detail in the following chapter. Morgan argues that even those who appear to be open about death on a verbal level may be quite anxious subconsciously or at the fantasy level. As can be seen from the different and contemporary attitudes towards death, there are other ways of looking at death, dying and bereavement. However, western society's attitude needs further exploration, not because it is dominant, but because it has been dominant in other areas of life (industrialisation, advances in healthcare and technology).

Aries (1974) postulated that attitudes to death over the centuries have been indications of a person's awareness of him/herself, as well as a degree of individuality. In his classification, Aries (1981) talks of four basic attitude orientations which he calls 'Tamed Death', 'The Death of the Self', 'The Death of the Other' and 'Death Denied' which form the death system. A brief overview is given here, but for a detailed account see Philippe Aries's books (Aries, 1974; 1981). The orientation of 'tamed death' was dominant until the Middle Ages, when life was poor, nasty and short. It followed that one was constantly exposed to death and became familiar with its presence. With such an abbreviated life, it was not common for young people to spend time, if any, preparing for adulthood. As shown by Morgan (1995), courtship was short, relationships were limited and education was minimal.

According to Aries (1981) there was a shift of emphasis between the twelfth and fifteenth centuries, when the individual became aware of himself as distinct from the community. Making this distinction, also meant that the individual fully ascribed to the death orientation of 'death of the self'. This was the realisation of the termination of one's life, one's personal death. Death became the last act of a personal drama, and at this point it was common to find tombs memorialising that life. Some tombs were placed in churches, and the different sizes probably symbolised the greatness of the person's life or memories being left behind.

In the nineteenth century, the above two orientations declined in favour of 'death of the other'. In this century life was viewed as having a meaning through relationships, (personal and intimate) and consequently death was seen as a loss of that relationship. For close relationships to develop fully, privacy is a pre-requisite, and so if death occurred in such relationships, it followed that the loss would no longer be a public event. In this context, death was no longer mourned as a loss to the community or as the end of life, but as the physical separation from a beloved one.

The twentieth century was seen as the period of death denied (Aries, 1981) where the death culture differed significantly from the preceding centuries. Here an understanding of the parameters of contemporary death attitudes becomes necessary, as they differ among cultures. The four major parameters to understand are: exposure to death, life expectancy, perceived control over forces of nature and what it is to be a human being (see *Chapter 2*).

Concluding thoughts

It is now being argued that death is perhaps not so much denied as claimed by Aries, but rather that it is a case of death being unfamiliar to most people. With the advent of institutions such as hospices, hospitals and nursing homes where people die, it means that the family members may not always be exposed to death within the family. When viewed in this way, death is being removed from the immediate family and witnessed by strangers who happen to be nursing and medical professionals. The argument that death has become unfamiliar would also suggest that people may not be comfortable with death, or simply may not know how to deal with its presence. If this is acceptable then it may also follow that people are fearful of death and do not even talk about it. The other factor to consider is that people are now generally living longer than before. This lengthier/longer life expectancy is due to a variety of factors, including medical advances and technology which have eradicated most deadly diseases, a better informed public with a healthier lifestyle and improved diet choices. Most children growing up in families may not encounter death themselves until they are in their fifties, when they have to deal with death for the first time and also explain it to their own children. This is probably one of the reasons why death is so difficult to come to terms with.

This chapter discussed the development of attitudes and suggested that there is a sizeable correlation between children and their parents' attitudes. If the parents have not formed an attitude towards death it may be even more difficult for the children to have theirs crystallised. There is however an avenue that could help with this apparent difficulty, that of education which influences the development and formation of attitudes. Education should teach and discuss sensitively the concept of death with teachers feeling comfortable and confident when talking about it. This kind of approach may not be a panacea, but it is a step in the right direction in that it allows discussion of a difficult topic to ensue in a controlled environment. Such an environment should also ensure that support (counselling) is available for those pupils who find themselves perturbed by talking about death. It may also prompt pupils to ask their parents about death and dying, which may be a welcome 'opening' for some parents, although others may be uncomfortable answering such questions. I believe this is already happening with some families, but needs to occur on a wider scale. Such openness may even be beneficial to the dying person if he/she can discuss his or her dying with the immediate family. The opportunity to bid farewell or apologise becomes a reality. One final word of caution, just as attitude formation takes a long time to happen, so too does attitude change. We can only hope to **effect** attitudes and then leave it for the individual to respond.

References

Allport GW (1935) Attitudes. In: Murchinson (ed) *Handbook of Social Psychology*. Clark University Press, Boston

Aries P (1974) *Western Attitudes toward Death. From the middle ages to the present*. Marion Boyars, New York

Aries P (1981) *The Hour of Our Death*. Knopf, New York

Bem DJ (1970) *Beliefs, Attitudes and Human Affairs*. Belmont, California

Devito J (1992) *The International Communication Handbook*. 6th edn. Harper Collins, New York

Elms AC (1976) *Attitudes*. Open University Press, Milton Keynes

Fishbein M, Ajzen I (1980) *Understanding Attitudes and Predicting Social Behaviour*. Prentice-Hall, New Jersey

Kastenbaum R (1992) *The Psychology of Death*. Springer Publishers, New York

Malinowski B (1965) The role of magic and religion. In: Lessa WA, Vigt EZ (eds) *Reader in comparative religion: an anthropological approach*. Harper & Row, New York

Mead M (1949) *Male and Female. A Study of the Sexes in a Changing World*. Dell, New York

Morgan CT, King RA, Robinson NM (1979) *Introduction to Psychology*. 6th edn. McGraw-Hill, New York

Morgan JD (1995) Living our Dying and Grieving: historical and cultural attitudes. In: Wass H, Neimeyer RA (eds) *Dying. Facing the Facts*. 3rd edn.Taylor & Francis, Washington

Nyatanga B (1997) Cultural Issues in Palliative Care. *Int J Palliat Nurs* **3**(4): 203–208

Radcliffe-Brown R (1965) Tabbo. In: Lessa WA, Vogt EZ (eds) *Reader in comparative religion: An anthropological approach*. Harper & Row, New York

Sears DO (1969) Political behaviour. In: Lindzey G, Aronson E (eds) *The Handbook of Social Psychology, Vol II*. Addison-Wesley, Massachusatts

Secord PF, Backman CW (1964) *Social Psychology*. McGraw-Hill, New York

2

A paradigm of death

Brian Nyatanga

It is impossible to imagine your own death, and whenever we attempt to do so, we can perceive that we are in fact still present as spectators.

(Freud, 1953)

The major academic disciplines have tried to understand the nature of death by compartmentalising it in a way that is acceptable for them. Psychology (Morgan, 1995) views death in terms of an end result of a process of suffering. Here the context of suffering relates to all the different dimensions that make up a person, and is not restricted only to the physical. Dying itself is characterised by suffering 'total' pain, ie. the psycho-emotional, physical, social, spiritual and intellectual (PEPSSI, see also *p.116*) dimensions of the person. The experiences people have in life contribute to pain, regret, fear of the unknown and guilt and all this amounts to suffering. Sociology considers death as the final phase of performing the different roles such as being a mother, a sister, a wife and/or a daughter to someone. This often provokes emotional reactions from the dying person and those of significance. Inevitably, where there is an emotional reaction, people need to be encouraged to **work through their grief** [1]. Philosophy views death as causing distinctive fears of non-existence, meaninglessness or extinction with

---

1   This term comes from the psychodynamic arena, and is specifically Freudian. Freud's basic view was that grief needs to be confronted, to be 'worked through'. Freud saw detachment or withdrawal of libido from the lost object as essential before the grieving person can re-establish or re-invest the libidinal energy with another person(s). Therefore, this process of 'working through' was seen as a prerequisite before the bereaved could move on into a new life (see *Chapter 9*).

no significance (Frankl, 1963). Finally, religion views death as a holy passage from this life to another eternal existence. To be guaranteed this eternal existence the individual should live his or her life according to the teachings of the Holy Spirit or relevant doctrine.

This philosophical position is fundamental in our attempt to understand why many people find it difficult to die and talk about death openly. This reluctance makes people conjure up different mental images of death, and so death continues to be viewed as a taboo subject, particularly in western societies. Aries (1974) claimed that death was so frightful that people dared not utter its name. Since Aries' claim things have changed in that now there is an enormous volume of writing on the topic of death. However the paradox is whether people exposed to so many writings go on to talk about their own death. While death is the only certainty in life (Field and James, 1993) and is one per person, it continues to be handled 'badly'. I do not believe that death is the problem, but the actual process of dying is. Considering all the care and resources available, dying remains a lonely passage in that no individual can live through the experience for another (Feifel, 1977). As well as physical, dying has psycho-social, philosophical and spiritual passages and the nature of these passages may be influenced by others. For example, in a social passage, what happens to the dying person is greatly affected by other people, who form part of his or her social world. Some of you may well remember the patient who 'puts off' dying until his son arrives from abroad or a grand-child is born. Is there a real influence or power from the son/grandchild or is this mere physiological coincidence. On the other hand, could it be the patient's power to control his own destiny in such a precise manner?

The knowledge or realisation that one is dying induces anxiety and fear. This death fear will be discussed later in this chapter. Dying is often viewed as synonymous with pain and suffering. This suffering applies to both the person who is dying and those close to him. Dying itself as a process can be avoided, and more and more people are asking for ways of avoiding or missing out part of their passage or transition when their own death is imminent. It is clear that you and I will die one day, but it is not clear that dying will be part of our life. For example, those who suffer a myocardial infarction (MI) or fatal road traffic accident (RTA), like Diana, Princess of Wales and Dodi Fayed, avoid the prolonged process (passage) of dying. This, however, would not be everyone's chosen way of avoiding the process of dying; people are now asking for more humane or controlled ways of achieving death. Proponents of euthanasia, physician- assisted suicide and mercy killing are campaigning for the omission or avoidance of this passage, presumably for those who are suffering. They all point out the degree of suffering experienced by the dying person. By ending the suffering and pain they also stop the process of dying. What this argument may be suggesting is that without the suffering, people would tolerate dying. This is worth thinking about, particularly for those of us working in palliative care, where death and dying are a common phenomenon. A fundamental point to remember about dying is that it often affects one's overall quality of life. Here quality of life should be seen as unique to the individual but may often be determined by others (like in a social passage), without finding out whether the individual concerned really wants quality of life. What needs considering is this emphasis on quality of life when one has a terminal illness as if this never existed before the diagnosis. The truth is that everybody has his or her own quality of life with or without a terminal illness, and this can be traced from birth to adulthood on a continuum. The problem with dying is that, even those who had not valued the quality of their life when they were well and healthy, are somewhat encouraged and persuaded to believe in and adopt a better or different quality of life. This is often set by the institution for the dying such as hospices. The question is whether the resultant quality of life is for the patient or for those in charge of the patient's day to day care.

When dying is avoided through MI or RTA, there is shock and disbelief in those left behind although, on the other hand, it may be seen as a blessing. For those who see it as a blessing, you could argue that they are trying to get rid of dying altogether as a precursor to death. Dying itself, as mentioned earlier (*page 12*), is characterised by suffering 'total' pain, the PEPSSI dimensions of the person. This holds true for the dying person and significant others who will be left behind. The realisation that dying causes enormous suffering forms the basis of the hospice philosophy and palliative care provision. Although the concept of a 'good' death seems popular in palliative care, Neuberger (1994) claims that this can be alien to other cultural groups such as the Jewish. It is worth exploring the notion of a good death using Bayliss's (1996) three categories. According to Bayliss, it is possible to have a medically 'good' death, which is characteristic of pain and other distressing symptoms being well controlled. It is also possible to have a naturally 'good' death, such as in old age. Here death is expected and is caused by the natural ageing process. The third category is seen as a religious or culturally 'good' death, where enough warning is given to carry out certain rituals before death occurs. This highlights the diversity of the notion of a good death. What is important is to understand an individual's way of viewing dying; their own individual paradigm of death and help them to achieve it. For example, what is considered a 'good' medical death might be perceived as 'bad' if it contravened cultural imperatives.

People tend to live their dying in different ways (Morgan, 1995). These ways are arguably dependent on three main aspects:

- the way people think about dying (cognitive dimension)
- the way people feel about dying (affective dimension)
- what people do when faced with dying (behavioural dimension).

The behavioural component as a response is largely influenced by the other two (cognitive and affective). In other words, behaviour tends to be the observable physical manifestation of the cognitive and affective processes as people interact with and react to their dying. Some of these reactions are well documented in the staged model of dying by Kubler-Ross (1970) and how to achieve an appropriate death (Weisman, 1972). If this analogy is acceptable it follows that people whose cognitive and or affective dimensions are not functioning, wholly or partially, would lack an observable congruent behaviour in response to their dying or that of significant others. It is worth taking a deep look at your own views at this point. For example, if you did not think of or feel anything towards your dying sister, your behaviour towards her dying would, most likely, not affect your PEPSSI dimensions, it would be a non-specific reaction.

This non-specificity is only an interpretation of that behaviour given the expected norms of your group of people or society. There may not be a clear-cut explanation for this non-specificity because of the differences in individuals. It is always worth thinking of cultural variations and their kaleidoscopic nature (DeVito, 1992; Nyatanga, 1997).

It is necessary when talking about a paradigm of dying to emphasise the social and cultural environments that impinge on the dying process of each individual. People's thought processes and feelings are greatly influenced and learned by such environments. In addition, there is a possible paradigm shift in response to changes in cultures or their key features. Cultures may change due to exposure to other cultures, the media, peer influence or direct contacts. DeVito (1992) refers to such changes as acculturation. However, while these changes take place, O'Neill (1995) argues that the rituals and practices at birth, marriage and during dying may not change.

A death system

Kastenbaum and Aisenberg (1972) maintain that a death system is characterised by two main factors, factual and theoretical. The factual aspect includes how exposed to death and dying one is. Also, the expected longevity of life may influence reactions to dying. For example, the current life expectancy of men in the United Kingdom is shorter than that of women.

The theoretical factors examine the way individuals perceive themselves as having control over the forces of nature, and also an individual's meaning of being a person.

Experience as a factual determinant of death

The experience that an individual has about dying may greatly influence his/her understanding and awareness of death. The awareness levels are discussed later in this chapter. Experiences are varied and the point to consider is whether such diversity has different influences on the individual. Consider an individual who experiences death in the course of working in a hospital and another individual whose experience was the death of a close loved one. The other extreme of the argument is that an individual with no experience of death may have a limited or completely intellectual/abstract attitude towards death. It is now claimed that people who have had near-death experiences change their attitude towards death (Greyson, 1992). It can be argued that a hospital staff member may be more aware of the nature of dying than a brewer, but more professional experience may not mean personal experience.

Another factor to consider is how long people live (life expectancy). For some young people being raised in a family that tends to live as long as 70+ years old, it is possible that their first personal or close encounter with dying will be in their mid-thirties. Their death system will be shaped differently from those people who grow up in war torn zones of the world or where people die from starvation, such as in Ethiopia, Rwanda and Bosnia. There, those who die will be both young and old. Life expectancy has been changing over the years. Lerner (1970) claims that at the beginning of the twentieth century life expectancy was not more than 40 years. Obviously, such figures reflect an average, since some people would have lived to over 70 years, while others died as young as five. Lerner (1970) claims that one other reason for the low life expectancy was that many women died in childbirth.

The way individuals view the world they live in and the extent of their perceived control of nature may shape their death system. Forces of nature play a part in our perception of death. One argument is that those who see themselves as having control over the forces of nature have a different view of death from those who see the forces of nature as having the control. By considering the following views, you may want to decide for yourself your own perception and attitude to death. One view is that nature is actually there to be controlled and used by human beings. Such a view encourages human beings to determine their own destiny and control their dying. You can possibly think of examples for this and in some cases nature is used to perpetuate the enjoyment of human beings. The other view is that nature is there to be respected and protected. The emphasis here is that human beings are already an integral part of nature. With such partnership the main aim is to bring the best out of each other. It is about nurturing nature in order for it to protect the individual. Those holding such a view may 'allow' nature to influence their death and so believe in fatalism.

Being a person

The notion of being a person forms the other theoretical factor (Kestenbaum and Aisenberg, 1972) that shapes a death system. In the field of palliative care, the central tenet of care is based on treating the patient as a person. Each person is unique, presenting with specific needs and characteristics. The question that needs exploring is what it is to be a person. A holistic approach to care suggests that a person is a complex whole with mental, social and emotional as well as physical characteristics. Reed and Ground (1997) argue that this is often called into question when one characteristic (mental or physical) is not functional for whatever reason. Of the two characteristics, the mental ability tends to influence or have more significance and dominance over the physical, even in pain perception, despite the evidence from the physical phenomenology of living. Reed and Ground give examples of mindless bodies such as algae and the vegetable kingdom, where there is life but which could not be classified as persons. This poses dilemmas for carers in palliative care and other related settings, where the minds of patients may be impaired as a result of their illness or their medication. It would be myopic to think of a person in terms of his or her mental activities, as this may lead to ill-treatment of patients as living objects. In addition to this philosophical perspective, the emphasis of being a person can be seen from cultural and societal variations. According to Morgan (1995) western culture places emphasis on the uniqueness of the person and his or her rights. Other cultures emphasise that a person is part of a whole, that is, focusing on a group or species of which he or she is a part. Cultural orientations lead the person to hold different views about death. There is another extreme where the person is perceived as having no meaning at all, calling into question the whole notion of existence of that person. Where a person is viewed as a whole, the social context of death comes into sharper focus (Morgan, 1995). This focus may determine the person's death system and consequently shape attitudes towards death. To determine a person's death system, there is a need to understand the basis of the attitude, fear and expectations about death. Such attributes are often an indication of the person's awareness of his impending death as well as his or her individuality. It may be useful at this point to explore well-known contexts of awareness in order to explain the points made above.

Although many authors have studied death and dying, eg. Kubler-Ross (1970) stages the process in psycho-social dimensions, Shneidman (1977) responds to challenges and Weisman (1978) is goal-orientated, aiming to achieve an appropriate death, the work of Glaser and Strauss (1965) on contexts of awareness will form the basis of the exploration.

Contexts of awareness

The contexts of awareness offer a sociological perspective on dying. Glaser and Strauss (1965) base their study on observing dying people and their patterns of communication. Glaser and Strauss claim that dying people go through four phases of awareness of their impending death, namely closed awareness (CA), suspected awareness (SA), mutual pretence (MP) and open awareness (OA).

In **closed awareness** the dying person is in 'total darkness' about his or her impending death. The relatives and healthcare professionals are the only ones who know and tend to engage in a secret pact of keeping this information from the dying person. There are possible reasons for this behaviour, including families being very protective towards the dying person or healthcare professionals being reluctant to say that death is imminent. It is also possible that the dying person may not be familiar with the symptoms of impending death (Glaser and Strauss, 1965).

However the notion of closed awareness itself is confusing or contradictory in that the two terms, closed and awareness suggest two parallels, or different states of being.

If one is aware, the interpretation is that there is some degree of knowing, although it is minimal. To be closed on the other hand would suggest total darkness, no awareness at all, no clue, complete ignorance as to what is happening. Perhaps less contradictory terms may be 'total darkness' or unawareness.

Suspected awareness is when the dying person suspects his or her poor prognosis. What he or she may be looking for is either validation or disapproval of these suspicions by family or healthcare professionals. It would not be surprising to find that most dying people would hope for disapproval, perhaps a reflection of the death denying attitude of the society we live in. The suspicion is often aroused by changes in attitude and behaviour of family and others, as well as treatment regimens. Treatment may change from curative to palliative, therefore focusing on the quality of life. The worsening condition often characterised by weight loss, is probably the single most obvious sign to raise suspicion.

Mutual pretence is psychologically the most challenging period for healthcare professionals. Glaser and Strauss (1965) claim that, at this point, the dying person, family and carers are aware of the poor prognosis but choose, by some kind of subconscious agreement not to talk about the impending death. Glaser and Strauss see this as a game of pretending, where all the 'players' continually have a mutual conspiracy not to admit openly the reality of the illness. There are many possible reasons for this behaviour, including emotional distancing from the dying person by the healthcare professionals. The relatives I have encountered in clinical practice, came over as being protective of their loved one. They felt that discussing the poor prognosis openly would result in the dying person 'giving up' the fight. The dying person often felt that the fact that he was dying was distressing enough for the family, without the added hurt and worry of talking openly about it. Therefore, in most cases silence on the matter was seen as a better option. While there may be sound rationale for this, we should ask ourselves whether this may mean missed opportunities to say 'goodbye' or 'I am sorry'. Silence may also exist because healthcare professionals protect themselves by not 'reading' the signals that people want to talk. Although it may be argued that mutual pretence is necessary to retain a modicum of emotional stability, this may also prevent dialogue about practical arrangements such as wills, insurance, property etc.

Open awareness is the fourth phase which exists when the dying person, family and healthcare professionals acknowledge and talk openly with the dying person. It is here that essential facts are discussed among the three parties. The practical arrangements or re-arrangements are made, for example writing a new will or changing an existing one. The dying person may be preparing for death, practically, but nobody will ever know what is going on in the person's subconscious mind. Although the behaviour in this phase suggests acceptance of the reality of their death (at a conscious level) they may remain unconsciously terrified of its occurrence (Firestone, 1994). Although it may seem super-fluous to carers, for patients to be accepting this realisation may bring with it fear from the knowledge of what is really happening or imminent. Constant interaction is needed in order to offer assurances and explanations to questions such as, care options, effects of medication, involvement of children and religious reaffirmation. Healthcare professionals may find it difficult working in open awareness as the dying person may request full information about their condition and illness.

Death fear

There is an element of fear attached to every death, even though people may outwardly be exhibiting behaviours that suggest acceptance of the reality. One argument is that the more aware of dying people become, the more terrified they are, intensifying the fear of death.

There are many terms that have been used to refer to death fear, such as death concern, death threat, death anxiety (Neimeyer, 1994) and these have been used interchangeably in the literature. What needs discussing is whether there is any difference among these terms. For the purposes of this argument, only death fear and death anxiety will be discussed. These two terms also seem to be the most used or referred to in the available literature. According to Neimeyer and Brunt (1995) establishing a difference between death fear and death anxiety has always been supported by those working psycho-dynamically, who link the experience of anxiety with the expression of unconscious conflict (p.52). However, since the psychodynamic approach has lost considerable momentum lately this has led to the theoretical basis for distinction between fear and anxiety becoming less attractive. When used in practical terms, that is, with tools or equipment measuring apprehension about death, fear and anxiety are equivalent, assuming consistency and suitability are ensured. It has to be noted that measurement tools are themselves subject to considerable debate, because most scales are thought to be unreliable.

The death fear that will be discussed here is what Tomer (1994) refers to as the anticipation of the state in which one is dead. This will also depend on the perspective employed to try and make sense of death. For this chapter, the perspectives of psychology and philosophy will form the bulk of the discussion, but before turning to these a brief look at gender differences with death fear will be considered.

Death fear and gender difference

It is thought that a difference does exist in death fear between males and females. However the nature of the difference is still poorly understood (Neimeyer, 1994). Several studies that have been carried out including Pollack (1979) showed that women are more prone to reveal their death fear than men. The discrepancy can be seen from women's ability or readiness to reveal their feelings more openly than men. While men may not easily admit or reveal their feelings, it should not be misconstrued as a lack of death fear. Men tend not to show their emotions easily, generally this is a western view but more specifically a Eurocentric view. Some studies have found no differences at all between the sexes (Stillion, 1985). What is of interest is that the factors that induce death fear in both males and females are similar. Leming (1994) identified nine such factors based on the impending death of self and the death of others. *Figure 2.1* outlines the factors that are intertwined.

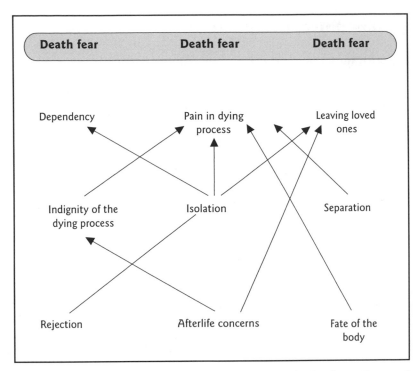

Figure 2.1: Factors that induce death fear in both males and females

The finality of death

There are exceptions to what is said above as not everyone will experience death fear. Leming and Dickinson (1994) claim that when BF Skinner was a dying octogenarian (at 86-years-old) he talked openly about his knowledge of impending death. He said that he was not worried or anxious as he always knew that he was going to die. There seems to be a degree of acceptance of the reality of death in this case, and this may also be based on the fact that Skinner had, in his own way, achieved most if not all that he wanted. His work was successful and being used by academics and students, influencing their way of thinking and behaviour.

Skinner (1904–1990) was a prominent psychologist who espoused the theories on programmed learning and behaviour modification using rats and pigeons.

Philosophical perspectives

The knowledge that we are unable to continue as a 'being' evokes a state of fear in us. Death itself becomes the ultimate threat to our existence, and realisation of such a threat brings about fear or anxiety. Using Heidegger's postulates, the realisation of our impending non-existence is a pre-condition for understanding our life and eventually a precursor to freeing ourselves from fear (Heidegger, 1962). This is supposedly dependent on the actual construction of death in our minds. For death to be viewed as freedom, its meaning must be established, seeing it as being something more than a threat to existence.

The other way of looking at death fear is to use Sartre's view, which is to see death as actually getting in the way of a person's potential and capabilities (Sartre, 1966). Death has the ability to reduce a person to a state of nothingness. Nothingness is like looking through a mirror of our meaninglessness in terms of our existence. Using Sartre's view, it can be argued that because people are constantly thinking of their death, there is a propensity to higher levels of death fear. Death in essence, reminds us of our past, or that which has been. If, for example, a person's life is not complete (complete being used in the subjective dimension) death may provoke a lot more fear or anxiety than in someone who has fulfilled his or her ambitions and other expectations, for example Skinner (see *p.23*). Where life is not complete, death is seen as an unwelcome, as well as an untimely interruption of one's life. This bears resemblance to the psychological perspective of self-actualisation (persono-logical) theories, such as that of Maslow (1968). According to these theories, self-actualising individuals tend to have a higher acceptance of themselves, less fear of any unfinished accomplishments and consequently a lower death fear. Self-actualisation may be a way of reinforcing a person's self-worth. Self-worth is about bringing out the real self by realising or achieving what a person really wishes to be. What one wishes to be is the acquired spiritual dimension of that person.

Psychological perspectives

Death fear can be explained by exploring theories that search for meaning (Frankl, 1963). The realisation that death is imminent, 'forcibly' makes the person review his perception, outlook, future plans and expectations in an attempt to rediscover a new sense of purpose in his life. In order to accomplish this, it becomes crucially imperative that the person has an appreciation of his relationship with the past. Frankl (1963) wrote, 'In the past, nothing is irrecoverably lost but everything irrevocably stored' (p.122). This is a clear demonstration that the past is the only certainty of a person's being, and true meaning can therefore be derived from it. Another way of looking at this, is to see life as full of potentialities that are in search of actualisation. Once actualised, they are rendered realities immediately, stored, 'sealed' and delivered into the past (Frankl,1963).

Another different perspective used to look at death fear is that of constructs (Kelly, 1955), where a person tends to construe what is happening at present in order to predict similar events happening in the future.

Constructs can be either core or peripheral. Core constructs are those belief systems that are deeply held by the individual. To change these systems and outlook would require a radical review (Tomer, 1994). Peripheral ones are loosely held and can be easily changed depending on the situation. It follows that death threatens the core constructs, causing radical changes to a person's outlook. When this happens it will induce high levels of death fear. What tends to happen is that the person finds it difficult to make sense of death, and Tomer (1994) claims that any event that cannot be subsumed often causes fear. For religious people, this fear may be to do with how their life on this earth will be judged in order to make the 'transition' to eternity. Eternity is the ultimate goal for religious people and the 'entry passport' depends on whether life on earth was lived according to set commandments.

For other psychological theories to explain death fear, the reader is referred to Neimeyer's 1994 handbook on death anxiety.

Concluding thoughts

It is evident from this chapter that there are many facets influencing a person's paradigm of death. The most prominent influences are rooted in past experiences with death itself either physically or conceptually. These experiences may have involved people close to you or have been encountered during a course of duty, therefore the impact may be different. Cultural and societal expectations tend to play a major role in shaping a person's paradigm. Such a paradigm is not innate but rather learned from individual families, peers, social and cultural environments. Holding such a paradigm enables individuals to afford symbolic significance to human mortality (Kastenbaum and Aisenberg, 1972) (see *Chapter 8* on the role of funerals). In addition to individuals holding their own paradigm, it is also obvious that different practice settings have their own perception of a paradigm of death. Hospital wards (in medical, surgical, paediatric, A&E, or orthopaedic) have their own way of caring for a dying patient therefore affording that patient a way of dying (hence a paradigm of death). The hospice settings are often credited with good practice because of the way they offer the patient a way of dying that is unique to that patient. It can be argued that hospices try to follow as closely as possible a paradigm of death that is preferred by the patient. The care that nursing homes give to dying patients may be different from that found in hospitals and hospices. One argument for the different paradigms of death is the influence played by the philosophy of care applied by each practice setting. What you may need to explore is why there are these different philosophies in caring for the dying patient in the various practice settings discussed above. It is well known that most people prefer to die at home, suggesting that the home setting affords patients a different paradigm of death.

The availability of resources, both human and material (equipment), also influence a patient's way of dying.

I have argued that death may not be the problem but rather the actual process of dying. There is evidence from pro-euthanasia campaigners of a wish or desire to avoid this process. The realisation that death is imminent, together with the meaning attached to it, often leads to a state of fear or anxiety. This chapter has used some philosophical as well as psycho-social theories to explain the possible causes of death fear. It is my belief that when there is increased understanding of what causes death fear for each dying person, better care will follow and help to make dying easier.

In our quest to understand why it is so difficult to die, the next chapter will explore the role of medicine and nursing in death and dying, considering death as the 'business' of others, how dying, which used to be a quiet family affair, has literally been taken over by others, by professionals and business-orientated people. The medicalisation of death is analysed to see whether it exacerbates or ameliorates dying and for whom.

References

Aries P (1974) *Western Attitudes Towards Death: From the Middle Ages to the Present.* Marion Boyars, New York

Bayliss VJ (1996) *Understanding Loss and Grief.* National Extension College, Cambridge

DeVito J (1992) *The Interpersonal Communication Book.* 6th edn. Harper Collins, New York

Feifel H (1977) *New Meanings of Death.* McGraw-Hill, New York

Field D, James N (1993) Where and how people die. In: Clarke D (ed) *The Future of Palliative Care.* Open University Press, Buckingham

Firestone RW (1994) Psychological defences against death anxiety. In: Neimeyer RA (ed) *Death Anxiety Handbook: Research, instrumentation and application.* Taylor and Francis, Washington

Frankl VE (1963) *Man in search for Meaning.* Beacon Press, Boston

Freud S (1953) Thoughts for the Times on War and Death. In: *Collected Works,* Volume IV. Hogarth Press, London: 288–317

Glaser BG, Strauss AL (1965) *Awareness of Dying.* Aldine, Chicago

Greyson B (1992) Reduced death threat in near-death experiences. *Death Stud* **16**: 523–536

Heidegger M (1962) *Being and Time.* SCM Press Ltd, London

Kastenbaum R, Aisenberg R (1972) *The Psychology of Death.* Springer Publishers, New York

Kelly GA (1955) *A Theory of Personality – The Psychology of Personal Constructs*. Norton, New York

Kubler-Ross E (1970) *On Death and Dying*. Tavistock, New York

Leming MR, Dickinson GE (1994) *Understanding Dying, Death & Bereavement*. 3rd edn. Harcourt Brace, New York

Lerner M (1970) When, why and where people die. In: Brim OG, Freeman HE, Levine S *et al* (eds) *The Dying Patient*. Russell Sage, New York

Maslow A (1968) *Toward a psychology of being*. 2nd edn. Van Nostrand Reinhold, New York

Morgan JD (1995) Living Our Dying and Our Grieving: Historical and Cultural Attitudes. In: Wass H, Neimeyer RA (eds) *Dying: Facing the facts*. Taylor and Francis, Washington DC

Neimeyer RA (1994) *Death Anxiety Handbook: Research, instrumentation and application*. Taylor and Francis, Washington DC

Neimeyer RA, Brunt DV (1995) Death Anxiety. In: Wass H, Neimeyer RA (eds) *Dying: Facing the facts*. Taylor and Francis, Washington DC

Neuberger J (1994) *Caring for people of different faiths*. Wolfe, London

Nyatanga B (1997) Cultural issues in palliative care. *Int J Palliative Nurs* 3(4): 203–208

O'Neil A (1995) Cultural issues in palliative care. *Eur J Palliative Care* 2(3): 127–131

Pollack JM (1979) Correlates of death anxiety: A Review of empirical studies. *Omega* 10: 97–121

Reed J, Ground I (1997) *Philosophy for Nursing*. Arnold, London

Sartre JP (1966) *Being and Nothingness: An essay on phenomenological ontology*. Citadel Press, New York

Shneidman ES (1977) Aspects of the dying process. *Psychiatr Annals* 8: 25–40

Stillion JM (1985) *Death and the Sexes*. McGraw-hill, Washington DC

Tomer A (1994) Death anxiety in adult life: Theoretical perspectives. In: Neimeyer R (ed) *Death Anxiety Handbook: Research, instrumentation and application*. Taylor and Francis, Washington

Weisman AD (1972) *On Dying and Denying: A psychiatric study of terminality*. Behavioural Publications, New York

Weisman A (1978) An appropriate death. In: Fulton R, Markusen E, Owen G, Scheiber JL (eds) *Death and Dying: Challenge and Change*. Addison-Wesley, Reading, MA

3

An overview of the medicalisation of death

Craig Gannon

Part 1: The background of palliative medicine and its perceived benefits in the care of the dying

A lack of definitions

In order to assess the role of medicine in the care of the dying it is essential to maintain an objective perspective, which can prove difficult. The relevant terminology is frequently misunderstood and applied inconsistently. Equally, the objectives and components of medical care offered to dying patients is poorly understood and misrepresented. Moreover, the emotive nature of discussions pertaining to death inevitably evokes individual or historical opinions, that cloud the issue further. These circumstances conspire to leave commonly voiced beliefs being ill-informed yet held with conviction. Clinical and personal prejudices make these mistakes as common within the healthcare professionals as the general public.

Literally 'the medicalisation of death' would appear to mean the practice of medicine as life is lost. This interpretation appears too limited to be of value. Intuitively the phrase might apply more broadly to medicine's role in the care of the dying and the bereaved. However confirmation is not possible, as Medical and English language dictionaries do not carry a specific definition of 'medicalisation' which must be constructed from medical, -ise, and -ation (Collins English Dictionary, 1995).

The 'medicalisation of death' was first used in healthcare literature in the late 1970s to describe the secular and institutionalised attitudes to death of 'modern' western society, with the accompanying loss of traditional coping mechanisms (Bevan, 1998). Subsequently 'the medicalisation of death' has been used inconsistently, reflecting neither its original meaning, nor even its literal/presumed meaning. It has been employed to deliver an air of authority to surprisingly divergent points of view. The spectrum of scenarios covered suggests that the phrase applies equally to non-medical as well as medical activity and can range from initiating cardio-pulmonary resuscitation (CPR) to merely the presence of any healthcare workers at any stage of a terminal illness or sudden death.

By contrast, this awkward phrase more consistently carries a negative intent targeted at healthcare (and not society's attitudes as originally intended). The very terminology conveys condemning overtones of imposition and overmedicalisation. 'The medicalisation of death' has not been used to describe the rapid advances in appropriate medical care for the dying, but rather an insensitive, excessive, or untimely intervention of the medical system, typically seen as burdensome in its attempts to prolong life. This confuses the picture. Ironically the area of healthcare most appertaining to care of the dying, palliative care, is seen both as the answer (McCue, 1994) and one of the culprits (Field, 1994; McNamara *et al*, 1991; Bradshaw, 1996) for the 'problem' of the medicalisation of death.

A discussion of 'the medicalisation of death' requires an appreciation of the complexity of possible healthcare input that may be judged appropriate in the time leading to, and after a person's death. As every case is unique, though a direct medical component may be needed in part, the objectives, the methods, and the level of contact required will differ vastly for each patient, at differing times of their illness. Once this intricacy is realised any umbrella term that attempts to cover healthcare interventions at and around death becomes meaningless. The differing medical (or other professional) actions cannot be grouped as if homogeneous, even for the convenience of criticism. Generalisations can never be made safely as to the wisdom of healthcare's involvement in the care of the dying. An equal right of access to good healthcare would appear central to a caring society. This right should never be stripped from a patient, but should remain true from the cradle to the grave (Clark, 1999).

It is worth highlighting that medical practice is not, and never has been, restricted to curing disease as traditionally thought. The medical mandate is dual, not only to preserve life, but also to relieve suffering. These two components are obligatory and fundamental to good practice. Once a disease has progressed beyond life prolonging treatment, the medical remit becomes solely to relieve any suffering. This reassuringly shapes an appropriate medical practice for dying patients. In the main there is little objection to the reduction of pain or other distressing symptoms via medical means.

Medical practice is compelled to respect the dignity of human life; this remains singularly relevant in its application to the care of dying patients (Latimer, 1991; Stanley, 1992; Beauchamp and Childress, 1994). Four cardinal principles are briefly described here and elaborated in *Chapter 5*. When considered together they can be used as an approach to most bioethical situations:

1. Beneficence: to do good, ie. relieve suffering and enhance quality of life.
2. Non-maleficence: to do no harm, ie. not to induce unnecessary tests or therapies.
3. Patient autonomy: to respect patients and their choices.
4. Justice: to fairly allocate resources to allow high quality care to all in need.

Thus medicine, although respecting and striving to preserve life, is equally obligated with dying patients, to accept the inevitability of their death (and discontinue any futile treatments), to facilitate their wishes to discontinue (or continue if appropriate) any treatments, and to maintain their comfort. This cements sound medical practice and should dispel the blanket negative responses that assume a harmful intrusion by medicine in the care of the dying. There are however described limitations to these principles; the potential for misinterpretation, the inability to cover the exhaustive moral content of medicine, and the lack of cultural sensitivity (Jeffrey, 1997; Davis, 1996).

Medical input to dying patients has differing aspects to consider. Though death may be a common end-point, the process of dying takes widely variable courses (see also *Chapter 2*). These require different levels and types of input from a variety of sources. A sudden unexpected death (eg. a fatal myocardial infarction in a previously fit person) will have no 'medical' need for the patient, but the needs of the bereaved may be incredibly high. By contrast, a patient with a slowly progressive but highly symptomatic cancer could have 'heavy' medical demands throughout the illness. Even within high levels of medical input, opposing philosophies in care of the dying are seen. The approach of intensive care unit (ITU) staff contrasts with that seen in palliative medicine. Both appear justifiable in their own setting, while remaining too different to come under a single label or a single judgement. The distinction stems from the essential 'likely benefit versus burden' analysis, which may justify the extreme measures employed to save the life of an otherwise healthy road traffic accident victim, but which may not be considered helpful to a frail patient with endstage cancer. However, the clinical situation is never absolute and rarely so polarised. The absence of neat distinctions means a reliable embracing of a single medical approach is not possible. Although the apparent inconsistencies make criticism easy, they in no way lessen the importance of a medical role when applied appropriately.

Medicine is not above reproach. Indeed, the hospice movement was formed to combat the acknowledged, but unmet needs of many patients dying from cancer, particularly in the hospital setting. By listening to these patients and their families it was possible to highlight the diverse and complex problems that faced them (Saunders, 1998). It became clear that these patients' healthcare needs expanded beyond medicine to cover many disciplines including non-physical interventions, eg. nursing, physical therapies, social work, psychology, and spiritual guidance. Contrary to the pre-conceptions there was an identifiable healthcare role and it appeared that a difference could be made to patients even close to death. Consequently, the hospice movement employed a multidisciplinary approach rather than the 'traditional' medical model, to address dying patients' needs and make the delivery of healthcare effective. It aimed to provide three main aspects:

- learning and science of the mind
- never-ending development
- vulnerable friendship of the heart (Saunders, 1998).

Though this included medical input, it remained patient centred (emphasising their inherent worth and dignity) above the role of any of the contributing professional groups. With this came a significant focus on the holistic approach, appreciating the important interplay between physical, emotional, spiritual, and social factors. These hospice or 'palliative care' principles have promoted the merit of physical and psychosocial well-being, not only in terminally ill patients and their families, but across all other areas of healthcare where they remain core values. Without such a philosophical and ethical basis to the care of the dying, unacceptable patterns of practice could develop (Latimer, 1991). The potential problems include; inadequate or unskilled communication of information, withdrawal of medical staff, patient labelling and poor healthcare.

In discussing the medicalisation of death it is important to review specialist palliative care, which is increasingly shaping healthcare for the dying. Specialist services have evolved from the hospice foundations to cover a broader remit in ever-greater detail. Three tiers of palliative care have been described that provide a useful outline to make the distinction between specialist and non-specialist provision (NHS Executive, 1996)

* **The palliative care approach** — promoting both physical and psycho-social well-being throughout all clinical practice; focusing on quality of life, the holistic approach encompassing significant others, respecting patient autonomy and open sensitive communication.

* **Palliative interventions** — non-curative treatments aimed at relieving symptoms or improving quality of life by specialists outside of specialist palliative care: palliative radiotherapy/chemotherapy surgical procedures analgesic anaesthetic procedures.

The presence of healthcare needs during a terminal illness is well recognised independently of medicine. National studies in the UK have revealed a need for increased palliative care services and resources (Addington-Hall and McCarthy, 1995). Impartial bodies such as NHS working parties have increasingly acknowledged the need for, and supported the expansion of palliative care services to provide healthcare for dying patients across the UK (despite the high cost implications) (DoH, 1998). Moreover, even the staunchest of critics of the medicalisation of death can admit that it has produced 'substantial achievements and significant benefits' (Field, 1994). These acknowledgements appear to justify, at least in part, a role for medicine in the care of the dying. This is also reflected in the rapid expansion of specialist palliative care world-wide (Higginson, 1998).

The benefits of a medical role in the care of dying patients

Healthcare plays an increasingly valuable role in the care of the dying. There are numerous and pervading benefits that can be identified as:

- accurate information that provides explanations and aids treatment choices
- active treatment of underlying or concurrent disease(s)
- relief from distressing symptoms
- reassurance and inspiring confidence
- respecting patient autonomy
- respecting public opinion
- empowerment of patients
- provision of emotional support
- lightening the 'burden' placed upon patients /relatives
- mobilisation of related disciplines
- bereavement support
- the advantages of specialist palliative care
- improvements in care for the dying
- additional indirect benefits of medical input.

Accurate information that provides explanations and aids treatment choices

Following a detailed medical and/ or nursing assessment, the cause of symptoms can be clarified (which may not be due to cancer as often assumed), and the patient's likely prognosis determined. This will entail taking an illness history, examination, and possibly investigations of the underlying pathology. This medical information can prove invaluable in directing treatment options appropriately and in providing explanations to patients, their carers, and other providers of healthcare. Without this insight patients are disadvantaged in attempting to plan ahead or make informed treatment choices.

Active treatment of underlying or concurrent disease(s)

Most would agree that medical input is appropriate at one or more points of a terminal illness, eg.

- at diagnosis of a life threatening disease
- at recurrence or disease progression
- at times of change in condition
- at times of physical and/or emotional suffering
- when death appears imminent
- at the point of death
- into bereavement.

However the acceptance of medical interventions restricted to specific events is not practical. Key times can be described, but a terminal illness is a dynamic process, without convenient distinctions. If assumptions are made, mistakes and missed opportunities will follow. It can be argued that not offering available and proven therapies would be unethical and medically negligent. As medical input can be expected at some point(s) of a terminal illness, ongoing follow-up is advisable, even if only to exclude the need for any medical input at that time. This ensures continuity of care and maximises the possible benefits.

Even during a patient's final weeks the potential benefit of active treatment should not be underestimated. Oncological, medical, and surgical interventions can prove vital in treating cancer, any associated problems and concurrent disorders.

This remains true for some patients with a presumed prognosis of only weeks or months. Such treatments at this stage may not only prove life prolonging, but also, and more importantly, improve the patient's quality of life. Even a few weeks of quality time may provide a priceless window to address previously 'unfinished business'. 'Active' treatments can range from simple antibiotic therapy for infections, to aggressive or more interventional options, such as; endocrine therapy, radiotherapy, cytotoxic chemotherapy, and intra-lumenal therapy (eg. cryotherapy of endobronchial obstructions) all of which can be surprisingly well-tolerated and beneficial even in advanced disease (Middleton *et al*, 1998; Hardy, 1996; Gaze *et al*, 1997; Thatcher *et al*, 1995; Maiwand, 1998). Patients would be denied these options if medical input were neglected.

It must be remembered that dying patients are not spared concurrent illnesses and have an enduring right of access to complete healthcare. Any coincidental medical problems will require appropriate attention. Good medical care must not be denied to terminally ill patients as their condition deteriorates, based on unsubstantiated presumptions as to the cause and irreversibility.

Relief from distressing symptoms

There is abundant evidence that a large percentage of patients dying with advanced cancer or non-malignant diseases endure a high level of unpleasant symptoms (Vainio and Auvinen, 1996; Conill *et al*, 1997; Addington-Hall, 1998). These areas of care need to be addressed. Medical care forms the basis of symptom control — the appropriate medical/ nursing input can alleviate pain and other distressing symptoms in dying patients. This can improve the quality of life, freeing patients to deal with the more productive issues of living and to face their future, even if limited. Pain, though perhaps the most feared symptom in cancer can be readily controlled in nearly all patients. The main reason for uncontrolled pain in cancer is inadequate management, not its refractory nature as often thought. Effective symptom control needs to be a continuous process to ensure that care meets the current needs, reflecting the predictably progressive nature of cancer and its accompanying symptoms as well as likely changes in responses to medications. For instance, up-to-date reviews of any medications will allow drugs that are unlikely to be still conveying benefit, or seemingly incurring side-effects to be stopped, and other potentially beneficial therapies to be offered.

Reassurance and inspiring confidence

Medical/nursing staff who are trained in care of the dying can provide an invaluable source of support. The wealth of experience and knowledge gained can inspire confidence in patients, carers and other healthcare professionals. It provides an objective evidence-based opinion to bring peace of mind to those who may otherwise feel like they are dealing with the unknown. The existing structure of healthcare services means every patient has 24-hour, seven day-a-week cover to provide equanimity. This is supported by specialist palliative care which has additional knowledge and skills in caring for the dying, and an increasing infrastructure to deliver it to all those in need. Some patients appear to require a medical presence, even without treatments, if only for the reassurance it can provide. At the other end of the spectrum, patients seemingly unhappy and unconvinced of their need for medical input may be similarly discontented should it be removed. Even patients who express concern at medical interventions to keep them alive when life has no meaning, may simultaneously be worrying about dying (Holstein, 1997).

Respecting patient autonomy

Healthcare is obliged to meet the high level of requests for care and support from patients with advanced diseases. Patients often appear dissatisfied when the active treatment options have run out. Such patients may demand further treatment, even surgery or cytotoxic chemotherapy, no matter how experimental, dubious, costly or far-flung. Treatments may follow on the basis of the patient's wish, possibly against medical advice. Patients with cancer have been shown to be far more likely to opt for chemotherapy with a minimal chance of benefit than their professional carers or people without cancer (Slevin, 1990). A recent study by Silvestri *et al* (1998) in advanced cancer patients showed a wide variation in their willingness to accept chemo-therapy, but with several patients happy to choose cytotoxic treatment for a survival benefit as little as one week. It may sometimes be the relatives (of incompetent patients) who elect for more aggressive management rather than members of staff (Moe, 1998). A demand for active input even to dying patients is shown by the large specialist palliative care caseloads, patients having requested or agreed to the medical/ nursing input. Not only do dying patients court medical attention, but contrary to popular belief they are happy to accept numerous invasive procedures and treatments (Meystre *et al*, 1997) and agree to toxic treatments for relatively little gain (Griffiths and Beaver, 1997). A study of recently bereaved relatives revealed that 17% wished for greater access to physicians' time and nearly 10% had wished that further attempts at life sustaining treatment had been pursued (Hanson *et al*, 1997). In addition, it appears that as death approaches, patients desire more formal rather than less formal medical care. In a study of their final two months, the percentage of cancer patients with their preferred place of care as home, declined from over 90% to about 50%, the remainder wishing for hospice or even hospital care (Hinton, 1994). Though this drop will reflect patients' fears of being a burden and the lack of available community support as much as any specific medical need, it remains persuasive that professional input for dying patients is necessary and desired.

Respecting public opinion

The belief in a medical role in the care of the dying also appears to be reflected in public opinion, considering the generous charitable support of independent hospices. Hospices form the largest charity in the UK (amounting to more than £100 million/year) (Saunders, 1998). With such a clear endorsement, do the public deserve to lose their right to seek specialist-supported healthcare once they develop a terminal illness? That would not seem fair.

Empowerment of patients

A key component of the medical assessment is to determine a patient's expectations and aspirations from any healthcare interventions. With this information, an existing knowledge of the available options, and a communication network to access these options, medical staff are in a valuable position to act as the patient's advocate. By providing information and support, and acting on a patient's behalf, it should be possible to facilitate a patient's choice, for instance their wish to die at home (Seale *et al,* 1997; Higginson, 1998), or their decision to discontinue cytotoxic therapy. An increasing but appropriate medicalisation of death paradoxically can reduce the medical treatments a patient 'has' to face. Similarly, the involvement of patients in their medical management may itself induce a sense of self-worth and determination, rather than being an imposition. Providing patients with a medicine to relieve their pain allows them to become the victor rather than the victim over a symptom that may have been a constant reminder and handicap to daily living.

Provision of emotional support

Medicine and nursing can provide psychological support to patients and develop coping mechanisms to help them face their diagnosis with the resulting uncertainties, symptoms, and losses. This can allow patients to find a level of comfort and spiritual ease that may not otherwise have been found. Though family and friends hold a key emotional role, the invaluable impact of external support during terminal illness and bereavement should not be underestimated. Frequently the presence of a trusted and familiar healthcare professional will enable patients to ventilate their feelings more fully, possibly for the first time, and without the fear of burdening family or friends. Also, an impartial opinion particularly if suitably trained can be a vital aid to reconciling potentially damaging family discord. More specifically, there is a high prevalence of depression in advanced cancer, which requires medical treatment as it is highly responsive (in >80% of cases) yet easily missed even by doctors (Twycross, 1997).

Lightening the 'burden' placed upon patients/ relatives

The healthcare resource structure boasts an impressive array of assets that can prove invaluable to terminal patients. Medical, nursing, social service and therapy staff can access equipment and allocate packages of care to a patient's home, or facilitate suitable inpatient care. This practical support can lighten the 'burden' of care for relatives (and correspondingly lessen the patient's guilt) or provide sanctuary for patients not wishing to die at home.

Mobilisation of related disciplines

There is a supporting role for medicine to the 'non-medical' care of the dying. Though the medical role may be limited a significant role remains in facilitating care from different professional or non-professional groups. A medical or nursing opinion may be necessary or influential in mobilising other relevant services, eg. occupational therapy, social services, or input from a patient's spiritual guide. Such multi-professional input can be the key to successfully caring for dying patients.

Bereavement support

Medical input can be instrumental in identifying the need, accessing the necessary support, or helping directly in the management issues surrounding difficult bereavements.

The advantages of specialist palliative care

There are numerous outcomes in the care of the dying that can be improved by adding a multiprofessional specialist palliative care team onto conventional GP and hospital services (Higginson, 1998). For example,

- better symptom control
- more time spent at home
- improved patient and carer satisfaction
- reduced overall costs
- increased likelihood of dying in preferred location
- greater information on condition

- better communication skills
- less likelihood of patient being admitted as an emergency, and less time in hospital.

Improvements in care for the dying

The formalisation of research and development within an academic framework such as medicine has led to better care for the dying. Medicine is constantly evolving, in particular the speciality of palliative medicine, which was only founded in 1987. Advances in palliative care have offered many patients a better quality of life through the control of pain and other symptoms, alongside attending to the different domains of their functioning. However there is a lack of awareness of these new skills, and existing expectations of established treatments are erroneously low (both curative and palliative treatment) with an inappropriately high acceptance of symptoms. Existing prejudices must be viewed with caution, particularly as they may be outdated and ill-informed. It is essential that advances are disseminated through formal and informal educational structures to make a difference to the majority of patients. There is still some way to go before all dying patients receive high quality care and improvements must continue (Addington-Hall and McCarthy, 1995; Addington-Hall, 1998).

Additional indirect benefits of medical input

Other unexpected benefits have followed with the increasing role of healthcare in the care of the dying. For instance:

- the donation of organs such as corneas, tracheae and heart valves (Feuer, 1998). This can deliver a great sense of worth to patients and their relatives that surprises many, as well as the obvious benefits for the recipient of the organ. Sadly, some have cited organ donation as a reason for concern, signalling the future 'inappropriate use of technology' (Field,1994)
- the high profile of palliative care has led to the propagation of its core principles to other areas of healthcare to reinforce the basics of good patient care.

Concluding thoughts

The arguments presented in this chapter set a clear justification for the role of palliative medicine, nursing and other complimentary interventions (radiotherapy, cytotoxics, psychology, pastoral and spiritual) in the care of dying patients and their families. What needs emphasis is that there are obviously differences in the way people view the role of medicine in death and dying. Critics of the 'medicalisation' of death continue to see fundamental flaws in such medical intervention, yet proponents of 'good' medical practice in palliative care will continue to justify the positive contribution made. At the centre of these contrasting views is the dying patient who may view these differences as making his own dying difficult. If we accept that each patient has his own paradigm of death, as discussed in *Chapter 2*, then the care we provide should bear no labels (ie. medical, nursing, psychology), but focus on helping the patient achieve his own desired way of dying. It appears as if the different professionals caring for a dying patient are primarily focused on defining their own professional boundaries and control first (a clear demonstration of professional ethnocentrism [Nyatanga, 1998]) before they begin to help the dying patient.

It is clear that the background arguments given have highlighted the perceived benefits of palliative medicine and dispelled the misconception surrounding medical intervention in the care of the dying patient. The next chapter offers an analysis of the role played by palliative medicine and focuses on the drawbacks of such input for the dying patients.

All references cited in this chapter will be listed at the end of *Chapter 4*.

4

The challenges of palliative medicine

Craig Gannon

Part 2: The role of palliative medicine

Analysis of the potential drawbacks to medical input for dying patients

There are many different areas of concern that question the appropriateness of healthcare interventions, ie. medicine during terminal illnesses. Although they are addressed individually they overlap, particularly the ethical aspects which touch all parts of healthcare practice. *Chapter 5* discusses the ethical aspects encountered in dying and death and so this chapter will only touch briefly on the ethical dimensions. Healthcare interventions include:

- the imposition of healthcare models upon dying patients
- unnecessary meddling in a natural process
- undermining patient autonomy
- generalisations of care
- the detrimental effects of good practice
- the potential for poor medical and nursing care
- an unchecked (or unstoppable) drift from appropriate healthcare aims
- the unnecessary and intrusive presence of strangers
- increased exposure to drugs
- the potential impact on survival
- the displacement of more relevant support
- abuse of a privileged position
- injustices in care.

The imposition of healthcare models upon dying patients

It is feared that the increasingly comprehensive involvement of healthcare with dying patients could generate or even impose patterns on society whereby people expect to die according to medical or nursing models. Once established such expectations of medical input at and around death would be self-propagating. This increasing 'medical' dependence could limit individuals' expression, and divert attention from the real issues of death and dying. There is circumstantial evidence to support this argument, with acknowledged changes within society in its approach to death. Members of modern societies find death and dying hard to accept (Field, 1994). Though medicine has been implicated as having a causative role, this appears unlikely as 'traditional' medical and nursing models are in fact constantly evolving in order to keep up with society's rising expectations of healthcare (Annonymous, 1998). The question 'has society led medicine, or does medicine lead society?' is impossible to resolve. The question is academic and in truth there must have been multiple influences for the observed changes.

An example of medicine's apparent influence upon the dying is the increasing institutionalisation of death occurring within western society (Hunt, 1997). Despite 50–70% of patients wishing to die in their own home (Higginson *et al*, 1998) there continues to be a shift from home to hospital deaths. Over the second half of the last century the percentage of home deaths has dropped in the UK from around 50% to only 26.6% (Higginson, *op cit*). Similar statistics can be seen in other industrialised countries, eg. France where home deaths dropped from 64% in 1964 to 30% in 1983 (Rogue *et al*, 1994), and South Australia where the proportion of home deaths has decreased continuously from 92% in 1875 to only 21% by 1990 (Hunt, 1997). Though historically the family doctor had an established and valued role in caring for the dying at home, the average GP in the UK will now only care for two or three home cancer deaths a year. These marked changes have fuelled fears of the institutionalisation of death within medicine and elsewhere, with suggestions that the shift may be an irreversible process (McCue, 1994), and if the trend continues, home deaths could become as rare as home births (Field, 1994). It should be remembered that these figures do not reveal that 90% of all care during a patient's final year occurs at home. According to Doyle (1998), the described decline in home deaths in

England has actually halted since 1992, with a possible 'slight increase' in home deaths. However as every patient's needs are different there are circumstances where a hospital would be the most appropriate location to die. For example,

1. The patient may want continuing treatment and/or investigations. Even patients with advanced disease need hospital admissions to exclude or treat potentially reversible pathology. This carries the risk that if patients decline rapidly, they could become too ill to transfer back home. It may be the genuine uncertainty of a terminally ill patient's prognosis that leads to unintended deaths occurring in hospital. Alternatively, the patient may not have reached a point in their illness that allows them to 'give up' on active management, so that they demand care in the acute hospital sector (possibly against medical advice). It is also important to point out that the nature and treatment of certain cancers, eg. haematological and lymphatic malignancies will in themselves make home deaths less likely (Higginson *et al,* 1998). In this setting, chemotherapy may be required even into the last month of life, and the potentially treatable acute complications such as infection or haemorrhage may subsequently be the cause of death (Hunt, 1997).

2. It is also important to remember the practical advantages that hospitals provide and not dismiss a hospital death as inappropriate without consideration of the individual circumstances (Gannon, 1995). Hospitals offer; diagnostic services, 24-hour nursing and medical cover, access to other specialist opinions, the flexibility of a large number of beds, and a location nearer for visitors than the nearest hospice unit. These benefits (Ellershaw *et al,* 1995) should be considered alongside the expanding provision of hospital based specialist palliative care that can deliver symptom control and support to dying patients in the hospital setting.

3. Hospital based expertise may be needed to deliver optimal symptom relief, eg. radiotherapy for superior vena cava obstruction (SVCO), or ultrasound guided drainage of loculated pleural effusions or abdominal ascities. Even symptoms requiring less technical inter-

ventions, such as nausea and vomiting can prove difficult in the domicillary setting necessitating admission.

4. There may be a lack of adequate healthcare/social support to allow patients to remain at home. Highly dependant patients may require 24-hour nursing care. Rationing of healthcare leaves such high levels of input rarely available in the patient's home. Similarly, resources may limit the availability or level of cover from community-based specialist palliative care services, prompting admission to a hospital or hospice.

5. Modern families may not be able to fulfil 'their responsibilities of care' (Field, 1994). This appears a consequence of changes in family and household structures, such as smaller family size, greater geographical spread, a higher proportion of working women, and the fragmentation of families through divorce, remarriage and cohabitation. This leaves deficiencies in the lay care available in the home setting. By contrast the need for lay carers has risen with increasing life expectancy, which prolongs chronic illness, disability and handicap. This point is supported by the fact that in the UK older men and women were consistently less likely to die at home (Higginson *et al*, 1998).

6. Patients may fear dying at home either for themselves or their family. This can lead to patients themselves seeking admission to a hospital or hospice as death approaches. These requests can arise from,
   • the fear of their symptoms being under-controlled in the home setting
   • the fear of being a physical burden on relatives should they remain at home when requiring high levels of care
   • to spare loved ones the emotional pain and memory of a home death (particularly where young children are likely to be present).

Clearly medicine cannot be criticised for colluding in these aspects of 'the medicalisation of death', which may actually result from good care, respecting patients' wishes, or resource shortfalls outside of the physicians' control. However, even hospital doctors acknowledge that, for a considerable proportion of patients, dying in hospital (more than a quarter) is not as appropriate a location as other places, such as home (Seamark *et al,* 1995). Good medical care should be responsive to the individual needs of a dying person and correct any shortfall . There is a need for better community support, community hospitals and local hospice facilities, to reduce hospital admissions and thereby increase the likelihood of a cancer patient's death occurring in a more appropriate setting (but still possibly not at home) (Seamark *et al,* 1995). The picture is improving. Present healthcare initiatives to develop specialist palliative care, in particular home hospice services, have been shown to deliver a higher proportion of home deaths (Hunt, 1997; Higginson, 1998). 'Hospice at home' services have rapidly expanded in the UK over recent years (Eve *et al,* 1997) but, despite their promise, they appear expensive (£5121 per extra home death in one study) and of limited impact with only one out of every three patients entering the service dying at home (Palmer *et al,* 1998). Nonetheless, the increasingly appropriate medical input to dying patients is beginning to redress the imbalance and significantly increase the proportion of home deaths again.

Unnecessary meddling in a natural process

Modern healthcare has been criticised as unnecessary and artificial meddling in the natural process of dying. At first glance there appears reasonable justification for concern. As a society we now label dying as a time of suffering, resulting from an acute or serious chronic illness or injury. This 'preferred' concept reassuringly implies that death could yield to medical technology, thus denying the naturalness of death as an independent diagnosis consequent to old age (McCue, 1994). It is implied that such beliefs reflect the latest technological advances in medicine having crossed natural boundaries to become detrimental. However similar criticisms have been levelled at medicine for hundreds of years and common sense tells us that present-day medicine will appear simplistic and even barbaric to future generations. We must not naively claim to have a control over nature that is anything more than progress along a continuum. Instead, irrespective of any approval or disapproval, we need to accept that roles have evolved for healthcare increasingly through-out our lives and then fight to ensure these remain (or become) beneficial. These roles for healthcare already extend from birth, through daily living (in disease prevention, eg. healthy diets, occupational health, child development, sexual/reproductive health and immunisation programmes), until death and into bereavement. A wilful denial of these roles discards any potential benefit from medical input, and when voiced, could discourage others from seeking much needed help and support. For some time healthcare has had acknowledged expectations broader than many realised. In 1958 The World Health Organization (WHO) defined health as 'not only the absence of infirmity and disease but also a state of physical, mental and social well being'. Though scepticism may remain as to the 'presumed and perceived' benefits of medicine's noticed expansion into everyday life (Field, 1994), the way forward has to be better outcome assessment to clarify the impact of medicine in these settings. This will provide a basis for supporting any truly beneficial measures and refraining from any interventions that cannot be substantiated.

Undermining patient autonomy

Throughout medical practice there is a fear that doctors and nurses (even when well motivated) may take a paternalistic stance that could undermine their patients' wishes. A medical presence could lead to patients enduring burdensome or futile treatment. However this need not be the case. All medical care is initiated, agreed, and continued by the patient or when necessary their chosen proxy. The patient is responsible for a healthcare presence around their death as at any other time. Medicine does not coerce patients to comply with treatments (excluding those patients detained under the Mental Health Act). If medical care is not required or considered unpalatable, the patient can simply ignore the doctor's advice. A patient can refuse any treatment whether burdensome or not. The declaration of Lisbon states that 'the patient has the right to accept or refuse treatment after receiving adequate information'. Although this is not the case world-wide, this right has been upheld by common law in the UK (Re, 1998). In France the patient does not have the right to refuse 'artificial prolongation of life', this privilege remains with the physician (Rogue *et al*, 1994). As discussed it is often patients that are pushing for treatments more than their doctors are.

The doctor's role in providing information to help patients choose or refuse available treatments enhances their autonomy. However any information is subjective, and a conflict of interest between physician and patient could corrupt this exchange. The process of deciding the potential benefit of a medical treatment over the potential burden can be fraught for physicians as well as patients, as a scientific answer has to be found without objective reference points. For example, a cancer patient's imminent death may not be obvious. As a result, aggressive anti-cancer treatment may mistakenly be continued. Doctors cannot be held responsible for not having all the answers. Better models to aid the prediction of impending death, would improve the data available on which to base end-of-life decisions in the future (Escalante *et al*, 1997). Regardless doctors remain obliged, ethically, morally, and legally to act in a patient's 'best interests'(Mason *et al*, 1991). This means that good medical practice dictates that knowingly futile or burdensome treatments should not even be offered, let alone administered to patients. Equally however, there are those within the medical profession who would opt for treatments without medical justification on the basis of 'compassionate' grounds. This can engender a superficial impression of being 'helpful' or 'kind' when responding to a patient's wishes (or pressure). This can rarely be seen as ethical when:

- there is no hope of benefit (ie. practice which is not evidence-based)
- it is likely to harm the patient both physically (treatment side-effects) and emotionally (lost time and collusion may prevent vital end-of-life discussions and activities being pursued)
- it is a clear waste of resources (Escalante *et al*, 1997) in healthcare time and drug costs from which other patients could benefit.

This balance of autonomy against paternalism is one of the most difficult dilemmas facing all healthcare workers, particularly those within terminal care. The recent emphasis on patient autonomy in healthcare delivery has proved invaluable in challenging the undue paternalism of the previously dominant medical model of care.

A patient's lack of knowledge or transient emotional state may mean that at some points of their illness they are not best placed to judge what is truly in their best interests. Definitions of autonomy typically emphasise the idea of a competent or rational person making choices for reasons that reflect judgement and understanding (Farsides, 1998). This will always contain subjective components that clearly blur its interpretation. Is it wrong to refuse patients' requests for futile and potentially dangerous treatments or an inappropriate admission to hospital (or hospice)? The distinction of right and wrong with autonomy and paternalism is not absolute but more about degrees and timing. This means black and white, fail-safe guidelines can never be produced although this should not deter any measures that could improve the quality of end-of-life decision-making and reassure many concerns. It has been proposed that incorporating a 'practical patient autonomy model' will both protect the conscientious doctor and be in the patient's best overall interests (Garwin, 1998). The suggestions include:

* Early in the course of the doctor-patient relationship, the doctor should determine and document the patient's wishes regarding limits to future medical treatment.

* The doctor should initiate discussion of the full ramifications of a proposed treatment. This should include any potentially negative impact on end-of-life care, eg. prolonged survival only in a comatose state or on life support systems. Studies suggest patients are reassured and not terrified by these discussions, but will expect their doctor to open the topic.

* Encourage the patient to formally nominate and fully inform a legal surrogate. There would then be an unquestionable point of reference should the patient become incompetent, from someone who was 'happy' to take the responsibility, prepared for the eventuality and properly apprised. This appears a more effective course than written advance directives.

* If the patient imposes limits on treatment that the doctor finds ethically unacceptable, the doctor should decline to act as the patient's physician.
* Similarly, if the patient finds the entire treatment plan proposed by one doctor unacceptable they should seek input elsewhere.

Autonomy's place is less clear once dying patients lose the ability to express their wishes. Involved staff may feel able or obliged to act as proxy for non-competent patients. Though this is a professional responsibility, there is concern that the patient's views may not be adequately represented. Care could reflect a single professional's own views rather than any consensus of good care. Some relatives may not feel sufficiently empowered to voice any opposition to 'medical' decisions, let alone anticipate it being acted on. In the UK the next of kin has no legal jurisdiction over a non-competent patient's medical management. The final responsibility for healthcare rests with the nominated lead clinician. To 'safeguard' the patient, doctors and nurses are legally obliged to act in a patient's best interests. In view of their unique position that combines knowledge, experience, objectivity, and patient intimacy, and appears a reasonable arrangement. However, it is not realistic or fair to suggest that this is flawless. Good practice would demand an agreement of all clinical parties: the GP/district nurses; hospital doctors; palliative care staff (if involved); and their family/significant others in accordance with the patient's previously expressed wishes. Clearly agreement may not always be possible as difficulties can arise from genuine differences of opinion or the practical limitations of reaching such a broad consensus.

The validity of healthcare workers as a patient's proxy can be questioned when disagreements occur within a team. The final responsibility for deciding best clinical management rests with the nominated lead clinician (typically a doctor). Delegation to another member of the team offers no advantages. For example,

* senior nurses (offer a different but no more valid opinion)
* more junior members of staff (might know the patient better but are less experienced)

- an independent clinician (unbiased but comparatively unfamiliar with the case)
- the team's chief executive (lacks the clinical knowledge and carries a financial agenda)
- the law courts (time-consuming, public, and emotionally and financially draining).

Medical advocacy or proxies will always be open to criticism, as any judgement of 'best interests' is open to question. A doctor's previous knowledge of the patient will never be absolute. Surprisingly, evidence suggests that family members are not necessarily a better proxy. Their knowledge of the patient's wishes may be equally limited, or obscured by personal opinion or grievances. Relatives can have misconceptions as to the patient's suffering (typically over-estimating symptoms) or may be poor proxies for reasons of covert or overt personal gain, eg. financial or social.

Generalisations of care

It is argued that any healthcare-based approach to the terminally ill will draw dying people into 'a system', to be processed as patients rather than remaining as individuals. This can only be partly defended. Inevitably in providing any service some generalisations will occur. And within well-organised teams of experienced and like-minded healthcare professionals, 'routine' areas of care will occur. This will remain true even as death approaches and no matter how hard it is resisted. Even within specialist palliative care which emphasises the importance of individualised patient centred care there have been criticisms of a pervading 'odour of goodness' (The editor, 1998). There will always have to be compromises. For example:

The rationing of resources: In offering a service to a population it will inevitably be tailored to the greater rather than the individual good. This is particularly evident on busy, under-staffed units such as hospital surgical wards where there appears little scope for the high levels of attention needed for individualised care of the dying. Even hospices usually operate referral criteria to target those with the 'highest' need, despite the benefits that could be offered to other patient groups. And within 'qualifying' patients, hospices are rarely able to offer individual patients long term inpatient stays (a rapid turnover is needed to meet the overall demand) or admission outside of normal working hours (when staffing levels are lower to save costs) even if potentially beneficial.

The maintenance of a workable service: Most hospices would not admit patients who were not already known to/ assessed by the service and normative precedents will hamper the spontaneity and flexibility of staff (McNamara *et al*, 1994). Tensions arise between the differing ideals within; the hospice movement, the constituent professional groups, the individual palliative care services, and individual members of staff. These ideals need to be compromised to reach common ground.

Altering a person's care due to their impact on others: A disruptive patient or one with an unsightly, malodorous or infective condition (eg. MRSA positive) may be moved regardless of their wishes to benefit other patients.

Education and research: A large percentage of clinical staff's time is devoted to teaching and research. Though this delivers benefits across the board, a conflict may arise when a patient with clinical needs does not get seen promptly because of a teaching session. This assertion should not be misconstrued, because the patient will always come first in palliative care settings. The nurse caring for or admitting the patient will be experienced enough to assess the needs and seek appropriate medical or further nursing help.

There are more worrying concerns that the consequence of generalisations could extend beyond the tolerable restraints of working practices. There is a fear that patients' deaths may increasingly be expected to be 'convenient' and eased towards a particular institution's or healthcare professional's concept of a good death. It has been argued that,

> *Making someone die in a way that others approve, but he believes a horrifying contradiction of his life is a devastating, odious form of tyranny.*

> (Farsides, 1998)

Unfortunately some hospice patients' needs do not sit easily with the service provided, though hopefully their care is rarely compromised.

There is evidence that hospice nurses manage less well emotionally with patients who don't fit their preconceptions of a 'good death' (McNamara *et al*, 1994). This is of some concern, as who other than the patient can define the 'good death'? (see *Chapter 2*). Further research shows that patients and palliative care workers differ in their conceptualisations of a 'good' death (Payne *et al*, 1996). The patients' descriptions of a 'good death' highlighted dying in one's sleep, quietly, with dignity, pain free and suddenly. The members of staff in comparison highlighted symptom control, family involvement, peacefulness, and a lack of distress. A similar study of Australian hospice nurses suggested that they believed a death to be 'good' if there was an awareness, acceptance, and preparation by all those concerned (McNamara, Waddell and Colvin, 1991). Difficulties can occur when patients only agree in part to the offered healthcare. Even though the refused component(s) of care may make up only a small proportion of the total care, it may be considered vital to the staff involved. For instance, hospice inpatients may refuse analgesia on religious grounds, or because of a stoic personality, despite clearly escalating pain and explicit advice. This is difficult to witness and may compromise other aspects of care (eg. avoidance of physical care for fear of precipitating more pain). This doesn't justify witnessed backlashes such as, 'if they won't have pain relief they shouldn't be in a hospice'. Such a desire to protect their patient's best interests, though well-intentioned, sacrifices the patient's autonomy. As discussed, the implications of patient autonomy are not boundless, however we must not be too conservative or restrictive if we are to remain true to the original individualised philosophy of palliative care (Farsides, 1998).

Generalisations of care to dying patients may leave differing religious, social or cultural groups feeling neglected by a non-specific service or, worse, one that appears to cater specifically for one sub-group. Hospices are criticised for catering principally for the white Christian middle classes. Indeed, in the UK 98.4% of hospice admissions are Caucasians which doesn't reflect the country's ethnic split. There is an important cultural sensitivity that needs to be integrated into any holistic care (McCaffrey, 1998; Tong and Spicer, 1994; Davis, 1996) (see *Chapter 7* for the cultural issues in death and dying).

Better training (including cultural issues), adequate staff support, and sufficient resources to allow flexibility in provision of care should minimise unnecessary generalisations. Conversely, generalisations are not always inappropriate. Though individualised care is promoted as central to palliative care, it co-exists with the 'generalisations' of evidence-based practice and ethical and professional principles. Palliative care must question the pre-eminent status it places upon patient autonomy if it is to remain above criticism of contradictions in care (Farsides, 1998). For example, there is an established opposition to euthanasia within palliative care, not merely based on the legal constraints (NCHPCS, 1997). However, a number of requests will come from competent, informed people who would never be swayed from their belief that euthanasia was right for them. By not acting on such requests, palliative care could appear only to listen to those patients' wishes which are in accordance with its own opinion. However the situation is not so straightforward. Although we may be sympathetic and facilitate discussion of euthanasia requests, there remain many cardinal reasons for opposing the legalisation of (voluntary active) euthanasia; patient autonomy is only one of many factors that need considering (NCHPCS, 1997).

The detrimental effects of good practice

Even within best practice inadvertent detrimental effects could arise from professional interventions. A healthcare role around the time of death may lead to:

The fuelling of false hopes: such as expectations of cure or unobtainable levels of symptom control despite advice to the contrary. This could impair the process of acceptance of the inevitability of death. These fears now seem outdated, relating to the collusion found within the medical practices of the 1950s and 1960s (Field, 1994). The withholding of information from a terminally ill patient is now rarely seen and acknowledged as bad practice (Buckman, 1996; Seale *et al*, 1997).

The fostering of dependence: patients may develop a dependence on healthcare in general, an individual professional, or a team. This could act as a barrier to communication within a family, add emotional strain or resentment, or allow family members to distance themselves from care and from facing the realities of death. This could reinforce and perpetuate a death-denying approach. However this need not be the case. As highlighted, palliative care values the role and needs of dying patients' family members. Appropriate care, besides helping patients cope better, should facilitate their relatives' needs and care roles, to aid both parties in facing the impending death more positively.

On a broader scale it is argued that there is a general and expanding dependence of modern industrial societies upon medical care to solve all their problems (Field, 1994), resulting in a reduction in the ability to cope with pain and suffering (Illich, 1990). This diminished ability for people to manage or to cope with their own health, appears to reflect industrialised societies' high expectations across various walks of life, with increasing dependence on identifiable organisations (eg. the council, their employers, the police, the government). Instead of marginalising medicine we should provide education to enable the general public to shoulder life's responsibilities, such as their health, and to relate positively to authoritarian organisations.

The hampering of established healthcare provision: there is anxiety that the increasing medical presence in the care of dying patients is unnecessary and hampers existing provision (Fordham *et al*, 1998). The involvement of specialist palliative care in terminal care has generated professional concerns within healthcare to do with the issues of continuity, responsibility and accountability. For example,

- the role of clinical lead becomes confusing
- increased patient uncertainty at conflicting management plans
- increased breakdowns in communication with reduced continuity of personnel

- the increased risk of de-skilling the non-specialists.

There are also worries of specialist palliative care's multi-disciplinary working (in particular the advisory role of specialist nurses) and a belief that any expertise is exaggerated or unscientific (Maddocks, 1998). However specialist palliative medicine involvement does not negate the need for, or undermine, any other support systems available to dying patients. The purpose of additional input is to complement and maximise the care on offer. Education and communication issues for patients, their carers, and other healthcare professionals is made a priority in specialist palliative care to minimise potential problems. With co-operation and good communication few problems should occur. It is worth reiterating that many studies have validated the role for specialist palliative care over and above existing conventional services (Higginson, 1998), and that the merits of specialism and teamwork are now widely embraced across modern healthcare. Specialist palliative care provides extra experience, knowledge, skills, and resources to deliver proven benefits to dying patients.

It has been argued (Morrison and Morris, 1995; Ellershaw *et al*, 1995; Grande *et al*, 1997; Barclay *et al*, 1997; Addington-Hall and McCarthy, 1995; Higginson, 1998) that some healthcare workers outside of specialist palliative care have limited awareness of symptom control measures (even the basics), possibly little information on when to refer and achieve reduced symptom relief (and other outcomes) in their terminal patients, suggesting a need for better training in palliative care .

Additionally there appears to be a general lack of clarity as to the remit of palliative medicine, as against terminal care, hospice care or palliative care (Field, 1994). This has serious implications in curbing professional co-operation. Indeed, the definitive aims of palliative care do not appear to have been universally verified. It is important to stress that clear and workable definitions of palliative care are freely available, internationally (WHO, 1990) and nationally (NHS Executive, 1996 and NCHPCS, 1995), while local guidelines can usually be obtained from service providers. Some details within these definitions will differ, and change is inevitable as palliative care adapts, but this mark of progress should not be viewed as a failing. There is a shared responsibility for specialist palliative care to inform other healthcare professionals (and the public) of their services, and all professionals caring for terminally ill patients to find out what specialist palliative care could offer their patients.

It follows that GPs and hospital consultants may be more critical of palliative care if they are unaware of the nature or value of (or merely feeling threatened by) the evolving specialist knowledge that overlaps their domains (Maddocks, 1998). Moreover, clinical care is only one aspect of the specialist remit provided by specialist palliative care. Education, research, advice, support and training would be lost if specialism in care of the dying were suppressed. Teaching programmes should ensure that the gained wisdom is passed on to re-skill non-specialists. To foster collaborative working, palliative medicine needs further integration into mainstream medicine. Palliative medicine's place can be cemented within medical practice by:

- ensuring palliative care provision within hospitals, for both outpatients and inpatients
- obtaining earlier referrals
- liaising with primary healthcare teams
- taking up formal teaching opportunities.

The potential for poor medical and nursing care

Though good care is the intention of any healthcare professional, there is a risk that poor care may be delivered to dying patients. Even within 'best practice' perceivably inferior even if still accomplished care will occur at the tail end of the spectrum. Studies have highlighted the need for better communication skills and better symptom relief in the care of the dying (Hanson *et al*, 1997; Addington-Hall and McCarthy, 1995). Healthcare professional involvement around the time of death also brings the potential for more untoward interventions. This may result from the subjective nature of many of the complex clinical decisions within terminal illnesses (as differences of opinion will occur) or less comfortably from a lack of knowledge, experience or willingness to follow good practice. Bad practice may be fostered by misdirected attempts to help, or direct abuse.

This ranges from genuine mistakes, including inappropriate therapies offered with well-meaning intentions ('the doctor knows best'), and spans to the coercion of patients for the personal gratification of healthcare workers, eg. research projects based on financial or career development issues rather than clinical grounds. A study in America concluded that some physicians might inappropriately use their medical prerogative to protect their professional autonomy. It appeared that extreme legal defensiveness could significantly influence some physician's assessments of medical futility, such that they would wish to pursue predictably futile treatments irrespective of the lack of any potential gain to the patient. In this situation, a conflict between the physician's interests and the terminally ill patient's own end-of-life decisions can be anticipated (Swanson and McCrary, 1996).

Medical care for terminally ill patients undoubtedly needs to be improved. However bad practice needs to be eliminated and not used as an excuse to condemn all medical practice and foil the good work that does take place. Medicine has to remember to respect care as profoundly as cure (Holstein, 1997). McCue (1994) argues that we need to prevent the overtreatment and overtesting of 'modern medicine's approach to the dying. This requires dissemination of the essential blend of science with ethics and the clarification of the limitations of available treatments.

The recent introduction in the UK of formal mechanisms to monitor and maximise the quality of healthcare delivered by the NHS should limit and hopefully eliminate poor practice. This includes professional measures such as continuing medical education, clinical governance initiatives, The National Institute of Clinical Excellence, and The Commission for Health Improvements. Alongside these improvements in medical education and research is an increased awareness of care of the dying, allowing the practice to continue improving. Sound, ethical research also needs to be a key component for this progress. Any research requires rigorous and independent ethical approval and patients must be fully informed and consenting. Many dying patients appreciate the chance to participate in research.

Progress is being made with the voluntary hospice movement being heralded as an example from which 'the NHS can learn' (DoH, 1998). Other shifts in care have happened, to improve the medical/nursing practice provided to terminal patients. In oncology a marked change in research methods, from a fixed focus on survival figures after treatment, to incorporate changes in quality of life, has allowed more holistic assessments (Gaze *et al,* 1997; Thatcher *et al,* 1995; Maiwand, 1998). Similarly Buckman (1996) noted that there has been marked improvement in communication between doctors and their patients with cancer. In repeated studies in the UK between 1969 and 1990 there has been a significant increase in open as opposed to closed awareness of impending death. As a result the patients and relatives were more satisfied with their degree of choice over place of death, were less likely to die alone, and more likely to die in their own homes (Seale, 1997).

Unchecked (or unstoppable) drifts from appropriate healthcare aims

The acceptance of medicine and nursing input in terminal care runs the risk that the evolving direction taken by healthcare may deviate from its intended or agreed objectives. It is feared that unacceptable healthcare interventions could thus insidiously become the norm. Some argue that this has already happened in palliative care with the loss of its original motivating spirit. Compromises have followed the encroachment of mainstream medicine with its technological imperative to investigate and treat, its professional (particularly medical) empowerment, and the need to conform to rigid standards and funding arrangements (Bradshaw, 1996; McNamara *et al,* 1994; Johnson *et al,* 1990). The original hospice philosophy disapproved of the care given in hospitals to dying patients (seeing it as burdensome and interventionist) and aimed to return patients to their own homes to die. Yet palliative care is now responsible for a great range of interventions for dying patients, and rather than increasing the percentage of home deaths, there appears to have been a movement of deaths from the hospital setting to another institution, the hospice (Higginson *et al,* 1998). This may not be as poor a reflection on palliative care as is sometimes implied. Instead it may represent:

- considered advances in available medical and nursing care, with subsequent improvements in dying patients' quality of life, but of a certain complexity to necessitate further interventions
- changes in society's structure (away from the supportive network of the nuclear family as discussed earlier)
- a response to the ever-increasing expectations of patients.

However it has been acknowledged that one of the challenges facing palliative care is to address the trend towards medicalisation (Corner and Dunlop, 1997).

The second scenario of healthcare drifting from its original intentions in its care for the dying is that terminal care is becoming marginalised within palliative care (Field, 1994). As specialist palliative care broadens to include patients earlier in the course of their terminal illnesses, there is the potential for a reciprocal decrease in the focus on patients' last days or weeks. This is difficult to dispute, and talk of 'the greater good' and 'equity' may sound unconvincing to those within palliative care driven by ideals of 'final care'. However the increased availability of palliative care should not necessarily have an adverse effect on terminal care provided that adequate resources are made available. Indeed, the rapid expansion of palliative care seen in the UK has had a significant NHS component, so a marked dilution of existing services to complete the broadened remit has not been seen.

The unnecessary and intrusive presence of strangers

Just the presence of healthcare workers could be seen as harmful during the period leading to a person's death. The involvement of 'strangers' could appear intrusive during this private family time. Patients and their families may feel obliged to disclose personal information and allow access into their homes. This loss of control, privacy and dignity could appear as yet another loss on top of the losses that typify a terminal illness. Continuity of carers with named key-workers can go some way to lessening this concern but although continuity is a priority in healthcare (particularly palliative care), this is not practical on a 24-hour, all year round basis. Even with the best continuity of staff this is only an answer in part, as people outside the circle of family or friends need to be involved.

Increased exposure to drugs

The expanding palliative care and medical presence in terminal care has led to a growth in possible pharmacological interventions with an acknowledged demand for rigorous evidence of the effectiveness of treatments (Ahmedzai, 1997). The increased use of medicines increases the risks of inducing; side-effects, allergic reactions, and drug interactions. Particularly feared are the highly toxic effects of most chemotherapeutic agents, which could appear to counteract their therapeutic value in the palliative care setting. However the picture is not that straightforward. A recent study of women undergoing high dose chemotherapy for metastatic breast cancer (with severe side-effects) did not demonstrate any measurable reduction in their quality of life as might have been expected, but afforded the patients the chance of increased survival and the prevention or delay of disease-related symptoms (Griffiths and Beaver, 1997). Another fear is that sedation could follow the use of drugs, such as painkillers clouding consciousness and impairing quality of life but, paradoxically, the opposite appears true. Good analgesia with morphine can actually improve psychomotor functioning, eg. driving skills. The importance of potential adverse effects from drugs is realised in palliative care, is carefully monitored and discussed with patients and if considered significant (or not manageable by other means) the offending drugs would be discontinued. This highly attentive approach should ironically reduce unwanted drug effects experienced by terminally ill patients, despite the utilisation of medications. Over recent years increased medical attention has led to a more judicious use of drugs, such as abandoning the use of the Brompton Cocktail (a mixture of morphine and cocaine, in alcohol, syrup, and chloroform water) (Ashby, 1998) and avoiding the previous 'heavy-handed' approaches to morphine dosages. Similarly, the importance of non-pharmacological interventions in symptom control is now far better realised to minimise drug therapies. Complementary therapies have an expanding role within palliative care, eg. acupuncture, aromatherapy, and art therapy. Specialist palliative care services and even cancer centres are increasingly providing access to complementary therapies as a core part of their remit (Clover and Kassab, 1998; Kite *et al*, 1998).

The potential impact on survival

There are fears that medical input may either hasten death or artificially prolong life. Reassuringly, there is no evidence to support these claims for patients receiving palliative care. Though the lack of any intended effect is highlighted within the WHO definition of palliative care (WHO, 1990) it would be unethical to run randomised trials in an attempt to find out whether palliative care did indeed influence survival (Ashby, 1998). Also, this patient group may still require acute medical interventions and decisions here are likely to effect survival. Ironically, some critics of the medicalisation of death see the artificial ending of a patient's life by an unnatural medical act, euthanasia, as a way of avoiding medicalisation! This is sadly seen by some as the only way to avoid burdensome life-prolonging treatment. But, patients can refuse any treatment, whether considered burdensome or not. By contrast many observers have confused palliative care with euthanasia (Maddocks, 1998), despite palliative care having dissociated itself from the practice (Ashby, 1998).

Of greater concern are the ethical questions raised by healthcare's inconsistent approach to nutrition and hydration in the terminally ill. On the one hand it is argued that dehydration can cause patient morbidity (eg. thirst) and hasten death (Craig, 1996), while others believe that artificial hydration or alimentation is inappropriate in the terminal setting (Ashby and Stoffell, 1991) as the limited data available suggests that they have no influence on symptoms or survival when death is imminent (NCHPCS, 1997). The use of parenteral hydration in the terminal phase could have detrimental effects (eg. fuelling false hopes, and being a physical 'barrier' for relatives) (Dunphy, 1995). The outcome is that terminally ill patients in the acute care setting will usually receive intravenous rehydration, while those admitted to a hospice or remaining at home would not be artificially hydrated (Dunphy, 1995; Craig 1996). Such discrepancies are hard to justify and do not inspire confidence in medicine's ability as a whole to act appropriately in the care of the dying. The reason for this quandary is the persisting lack of definitive research and until this is found it is likely that medicine will continue to divide into two camps of 'standard' management. In the meantime, we must admit our uncertainty, make individualised decisions, not prejudgements, remembering to elicit and treat any reversible causes of dehydration (eg. hypercalcaemia), and be responsive to the wishes of the patient and their family (Dunphy, 1995; Dunlop *et al*, 1995). A recent consensus document summarises the current knowledge base to provide a framework for good practice (NCHPCS, 1997). The way forward is ongoing research to provide sufficiently substantive data to unite medicine in its management of terminal dehydration.

A similar divergence of opinion and practice is seen in another highly emotive area, cardiopulmonary resuscitation (CPR) for the terminally ill. Though great strides have been made in recent years (BMA and RCN, 1993; NCHPCS, 1997) with better understanding and practice following consensus statements, there is still considerable variance in common practice. In the hospital setting, irrespective of their condition, patients will remain for resuscitation from the point of their admission until some later time when the issue of whether to resuscitate may (or may not) be discussed. By contrast, patients admitted to a hospice would not even be considered for resuscitation as standard practice, equally it would rarely be discussed or documented (Dunphy, 1997). Considering these two patient groups, the 'opt in' resuscitation policy seen in hospitals against the 'opt out' policy common to hospices would seem wholly appropriate for the majority of cases. There is good evidence that CPR in the setting of advanced metastatic cancer is unlikely to be successful. However a blanket approach is easily open to challenge. Two thirds of all deaths in the UK occur in hospital. This includes patients with advanced cancer, so it is likely that there will be many futile attempts at resuscitation within hospitals. And hospices are now admitting patients far earlier in the course of their illness when resuscitation could be of value, yet hospices do not normally have the skilled staff or equipment to even offer advanced life support. In addition, as the issue of CPR is rarely discussed within hospices, patients may be missed who wish for, and not unreasonably, might be expecting resuscitation in a healthcare setting. These issues are well recognised and implementation of the mentioned guidelines should continue to improve practice. Similar attention must also be given to terminally ill patients in the domicillary setting where doctor-and-patient agreed anticipatory decisions on resuscitation need to be recorded and communicated to any designated nursing or medical cover (eg. GP deputising services), ambulance services and, of course, all carers.

The role of sedative medications can also take on a specific ethical perspective. When death approaches with distressing symptoms that appear refractory to all measures, the use of sedation as a means of symptom control may have to be considered. This is a difficult area. A dangerous precedent can appear to be set whatever is done, with medicine over-stepping its boundaries if sedation is prescribed, or acting barbarically if relief is denied an imminently dying patient by withholding sedatives. The use of sedation is overrun with difficulties, such as confirming the refractory nature of the symptom(s) and the apparent endstage of the patient's illness, as well as achieving a consensus of all involved parties as mentioned earlier (the patient, the family/carers, and other healthcare professionals). Distinctions in practice can be seen. It is normal in palliative care to use sedative medications to relieve the symptoms of terminal restlessness during a patient's final hours or days. However sedating a patient who is not dying to the point of coma for an indefinite period to relieve refractory symptoms is not part of normal palliative care (Ashby, 1998). To summarise:

* Following appropriate assessment when sedation is still considered unequivocally necessary, its conservative use can be considered ethical within the realms of the double effect doctrine. This states that a bad effect such as a patient's death may be permissible if it is not intended and occurs as a side-effect of a beneficial action (Thorns, 1998). *Chapter 5* discusses this doctrine in more detail, but it is important to stress that the doctrine of double effect must be applied with care and accuracy.

The displacement of more relevant support

It is argued that the presence of healthcare professionals in the care of dying patients can divert attention from more appropriate channels of support. Though possible, this need not be the case, and the opposite may be true. Undoubtedly for a number of patients, lay carers and non-healthcare professionals will be better placed to comfort them when death draws close and the 'traditional' role of medicine is reduced. Palliative care sets out to utilise all potential sources of support in order to benefit the patient, which may not include any ongoing medical input. It is increasingly common for specialist palliative care teams to refer patients back when a specific need can no longer be identified. The patient is encouraged to follow the most suitable line(s) of support, eg. family, friends, spiritual and/or self-help groups. There should never be any routine healthcare provision to dying patients. Medicine's regard for the role of non-professional carers in supporting terminally ill patients is seen in the ongoing research into the collective wisdom of lay people who were familiar with dying and death (Donnelly, 1999).

Abuse of a privileged position

A drawback of a close professional relationship in an emotive area such as dying is that it can foster the feeling within individual staff or healthcare teams that they must be indispensable. Healthcare staff may consciously or sub-consciously take on more than their training or skills allow, preventing patients from benefiting from more appropriate lines of help. For example, problems can occur when healthcare workers feel obliged to advise on unfamiliar diseases or drugs (without adequate knowledge) or to intervene in difficult family situations, eg. marital discord (without sufficient training). This appears particularly relevant within specialist palliative care where the 'holistic' remit seems without boundaries. Despite specialist palliative care's multidisciplinary base, continuity of care is typically provided by a single person in a single discipline (usually nursing), endeavouring to meet a vast scope of needs. An understandable but not defendable self-belief can develop, with an individual staff member or professional group seeing themselves as 'all knowledgeable' in the care of the dying. To avoid this it is necessary to improve healthcare workers awareness of professional and ethical boundaries, as well as providing adequate staff support and supervision in a multidisciplinary context.

Injustices in care

Injustices in the provision of care, whether real or perceived, may follow the further development of healthcare input to dying patients. Inconsistencies can be seen in the provision and the delivery of specialist (and non-specialist) palliative care that occurs from one region to the next. For example, inadequacies in the approach to dying patients still remain evident within the hospital and community settings (Field, 1994). Corresponding inequities can be seen in specialist palliative care provision. Differences in which diagnoses qualify for input, the stage of the illness, and the range of specialist palliative care services that patients are likely to receive can vary dramatically. Even within the UK, the birthplace of the modern hospice movement, there are noticeable discrepancies in the provision of hospice beds across the country (Eve *et al*, 1997), with regional variations ranging from 34 to 65 beds per million population in 1994. In 1995/96 the number of patients with malignant disease gaining access to hospice beds varied from 18% in Trent Region to 30% in the North West Region (NCHPCS, 1997).

A gaze into other surrounding issues in palliative care

Another discrepancy is that while cancer is responsible for a quarter of all deaths in Britain, it accounts for more than 95% of specialist palliative care workload (Eve *et al*, 1997). Yet there is evidence that hospice style care is needed for many patients with illnesses other than cancer. Studies have shown that during the last year of a non-malignant illness, symptoms are prolonged and common with a similar symptom prevalence to malignant illnesses (eg. pain in about half). This patient group receives less supportive care, eg. they are less well-informed by their healthcare professionals (Addington-Hall, 1998). Patients with non-malignant diseases appear greatly disadvantaged in accessing hospice services. There are many factors that have combined to give the sketchy, cancer specific picture found in UK hospice care. These include:

* The original focus of the pioneers in palliative care was to improve the quality of care to end-stage cancer patients. Hospices did not set out or claim to 'tackle all the problems of terminal care' (Saunders, 1994). This original remit has had a carry-over effect on subsequent services. However forty years on hospice services are looking ahead as to how to use best the knowledge that they have gained.

* The resulting evidence base has been cancer-centred and not necessarily applicable to other diseases just because death may be close. This has to be the prompt for more research into symptom control of end-stage non-malignant illnesses. In the meantime we must use the experience we have from treating cancer patients for treating non-cancer patients (optimally with the support of the patient's other specialists, eg. a cardiologist in the case of heart failure).

* The predominantly charitable nature of hospice funding has dictated the direction of care. The success of specific fund-raising for an emotive disease such as cancer has determined a disease specific service in areas of high charitable donations. Increased public awareness of the needs of less high profile diseases and more NHS funding is necessary to redress the imbalance.

* As an evolving area of healthcare, 'baseline' palliative care services are still being established, leaving gaps yet to be filled. In the UK NHS measures, though nominally cancer orientated, are in place that should continue to improve availability of specialist palliative care (NHS Executive, 1995), with demands that the benefits should extend beyond cancer patients (NHS Executive, 1996).

* Palliative care services are directed towards patients with specific indications for specialist input. This leaves nearly 50% of cancer patients not receiving hospice input as it is

not needed (Eve *et al*, 1997). Increasingly palliative care services are providing 'open access' for patients with advanced disease irrespective of their diagnosis without the anticipated influx of non-malignant patients. Despite the unquestionable areas of overlap within terminal illnesses due to malignant and benign causes, it appears that a larger percentage of patients with advanced cancer need specialist palliative care, relative to other advanced diseases. There are numerous reasons. Malignant diseases deliver a more predictable decline to identify an anticipatory terminal phase with a short prognosis. The symptom picture tends to be faster changing, more distressing (including more pain) and less predictable with overlapping aetiologies. This leads to the 'cancer fog' which necessitates the multi-professional input characteristic of specialist palliative care. By contrast, advanced non-malignant diseases generally have a less predictable prognosis at the 'terminal' phase (with sudden deaths or prolonged survivals), a more stable (but prolonged) and predictable symptom picture, and one that can be more clearly linked to the underlying pathology (eg. dyspnoea in heart failure) (Addington-Hall, 1998). Though dying from a non-malignant disease presents an equally distressing picture, equally in need of non-specialist palliative care, such patients often warrant ongoing specialist disease modifying treatment, eg. cardiology input for end-stage heart failure. Addington-Hall claims that this should be informed by palliative care principles alongside specialist palliative care when particularly complex problems are encountered. These patients would be appropriate for specialist palliative care once their underlying condition has advanced to become refractory to available therapies and/or the patient with end-stage disease has made an informed decision not to pursue further active management.

Concern also surrounds hospice care's apparent 'insistence' on quality at the expense of quantity. This has led to the suggestion that, 'the five star service for the select few provided by hospice organisations should be replaced by three star care for all' (Field, 1994). It seems puzzling that high quality care can now be grounds for criticism. Instead of sinking to the lowest common denominator, it would appear a more prudent objective to improve the care provided by supplying the best service to everyone who needs it.

Unfortunately inequalities in the provision of specialist care do still occur and need to be rectified. There is increasing awareness of the needs of patients dying from non-malignant diseases, the lack of culturally sensitive services (see *Chapter 7*), and the absence of specialist teams in some areas. These issues are now acknowledged as priorities to be addressed by those in palliative care (Corner and Dunlop, 1995; Higginson, 1998). Subsequently, there is a conscious effort through the work of the Department of Health (DoH, 1998) to work towards delivering high quality, appropriate 'palliative care for all'.

Concluding thoughts

An enduring right of access to good healthcare is central to a caring society. Within this the discipline of medicine sets out to relieve suffering as well as cure disease. By the time a patient has an advanced disease that has progressed beyond cure, the focus of their medical input will shift to centre on the relief of suffering. Though at odds with the traditional view of medicine, the value of this medical input in caring for the terminally ill could not be more relevant; delivering benefits in both quantitative survival and quality of remaining life. Allowing for the contrasts in different patients' needs and the scope of healthcare available there appears merit in a tailored medical input to the care of the dying. Though the palpable medical role may be limited there will remain a significant role for medicine in supporting the different professional groups. However, dying patients do not need a compulsory medical input, just its consideration and availability when an agreed and achievable benefit can be identified. Medicine does not claim an extraordinary juris-diction over dying people, nor can it singularly offer a better death, but neither can it be absent (Holstein, 1997).

Unfortunately, numerous drawbacks can be identified in the present delivery of medical care to the terminally ill. Rather than prompting the rejection of medicine and all it offers, this should serve as the necessary spur to improve the quality of medical input to the dying. The future lies in continued education of the medical community to understand the value of care and transform death back onto a human scale. Alongside this, an increased awareness and integration of medical ethics into everyday practice is imperative. Ethics can secure the quality of care, for example formulating the necessary condemnation of futile or burdensome therapies offered only to be doing everything possible, rather than doing the right thing.

Similarly nursing and other professions, such as physical therapies and social work are ideally positioned to have a dramatic impact on patients by considering healthcare issues within the context of a person's activities of daily living. This attention to individual functioning further refines quality of life issues to complement other provided care. Quality of life becomes the key goal as death approaches, and the distinctions between the different healthcare professionals' roles and non-healthcare interventions inevitably blur. This overlap should be seen as an opportunity for flexibility to provide more extensive and appropriate benefits to patients.

Field (1994) makes the point that members of modern societies find the naturalness of death and dying hard to accept. This avoidance by society of the inevitability of death appears to be a coping mechanism for which medicine cannot be held accountable. Medicine may offer life-prolonging treatment and though death may be postponed, it can never be evaded. Life-prolonging treatment is not restricted to the care of the dying, but an everyday occurrence in medicine. Even simple infections could be fatal without appropriate antibiotic treatment. This applies equally to patients with far-advanced disease. The question is not whether the pursuit of life-prolonging treatment is right or wrong in the care of terminally ill patients, but when might it be right or wrong. Medicine retains a legal and moral duty to provide treatment options that are in the patient's best interests. This responsibility for deciding appropriate health-care is a clinical issue that cannot adequately be abdicated to others. However whether to accept offered treatments remains the decision of the patient alone. It is not for relatives, physicians, nurses or society to impose their value system on an individual simply because they have become terminally ill. When viewed like this, it is clear to see why it is difficult to die, let alone to make decisions that are not only in the best interest of the dying patient but also the family in bereavement. A person's worth and basic rights are not lessened in any way by an advancing disease.

As each person is unique, so too is his or her death. Although parts may be shared, as bystanders we are unlikely to see more than a glimpse of the true picture, each of us from a different perspective. The experience is based on the disease, the personality, the available support and prior life events, in particular any dealings with death. The perceptions will be constantly changing as each new moment has its own impact. These are some of the factors that help shape the dying person's paradigm of death (see *Chapter 2*). There will also be additional external influences from society and a patient's cultural background. Consequently, each dying patient's requirements will be unique, though these are likely to include some degree of medical input at some time. This medical need should never be presumed or denied, but assessed and delivered when required as part of the 'total care' of patients with terminal illnesses. This should ensure that any 'medicalisation of death' is seen as a valued component of care. Just as medicine should not dictate the path of dying, philosophers and sociologists should not expect to impose their belief systems to turn terminal patients away from the benefits of medicine. Instead, a collaborative approach would seem to be in the patients' and society's best interests (McCue, 1994). This is the ideal embodied in specialist palliative care's multi-disciplinary approach, which looks to all avenues for guidance on how to deliver the best care to dying patients.

Specialist palliative care integrates medicine, nursing, social work, pastoral/spiritual care, physiotherapy, occupational therapy, pharmacy and other related disciplines. The availability of specialist palliative care is now considered a prerequisite component of cancer care in the UK following the Calman-Hine report of 1995. There is increasing support for this input to be available to all far advanced diseases. The blend of disciplines allows palliative care to provide an increasingly holistic approach for those with an identifiable need who request it. Though medical input is a significant component of this care, the term 'medicalisation' appears to undervalue such a broad mix of skills that combine to deliver patient-centred support incorporating physical, psychological, spiritual, and social elements. Palliative care is expanding rapidly, with increasing expectations from specialist and non-specialist healthcare to dying patients. Though this input cannot escape the label 'medicalisation', hopefully it may with time evoke a more positive use of the term.

Unfortunately theory and practice do not always meet, and many problems are acknowledged within palliative care provision. This is not surprising considering the emotive mix of complex clinical, social and ethical dilemmas within care of the dying and the high resource implications that follow. However they remain key areas to address within palliative care, which constantly aims to improve the quality of care provided to dying patients. Despite the actual and potential problems, the proven benefit from palliative care interventions generates overwhelming support for healthcare involvement in the care of the dying on a pragmatic basis.

There are no generalisations possible in dealing with death and dying. The value of philosophical, sociological, spiritual and medical/nursing models of death lies in aiding research and academic understanding. It would be a mistake to hide behind such banners and claim that the existing care of the dying is good or bad according to any one system. Any single-mindedness may divert possible support from the attentiveness and loving relationships central to life's end. It is easy to criticise the existing healthcare model of input to dying patients. However, no 'system' will ever do justice to the complex, dynamic, intensive, numerous, and at times irresolute needs of the terminally ill. We must resist falling in with the criticisms of healthcare interventions that are freely voiced without proposing much in the way of practical alternatives. It would be unwise to repeat the mistakes of the past and return to a nihilistic state, undoing all the progress that has already been made. We should acknowledge that dying is not always open to solutions. Equally, we should endeavour to do what we can and not abandon people as their death approaches. This way guarantees dignity for the dying individual.

References

Addington-Hall J (1998) Palliative care in non-malignant disease. *Palliat Care Today* **7**(1): 10–11

Addington-Hall J, McCarthy M (1995) Dying from cancer: Results of a national population based investigation. *Palliat Med* **9**: 295–305

Ahmedzai S (1997) Five year threads (editorial). *Prog in Palliat Care* **5**: 235–7

Anonymous (1998) *Maintaining Good Medical Practice*. The General Medical Council, London: July

Ashby M (1998) Palliative care, death causation, public policy and the law. *Prog in Palliat Care* **6**(3): 69–77

Ashby M, Stoffel B (1991) Therapeutic ratio and defined phases: proposal of ethical framework for palliative care. *Br Med J* **302**: 1322–24

Barclay SIG, Todd CJ, Grade GE *et al* (1997) How common is medical training in palliative care? A postal survey of general practitioners. *Br J Gen Pract* **47**: 800–805

Beauchamp T, Childress J (1994) *The Principles of Biomedical Ethics*. 4th edn. Oxford University Press, Oxford

Bevan D (1998) Death, dying and inequality care. *J Prac Development* **7**(1): Dec

BMA, RCN (1993) *Decisions relating to cardiopulmonary resuscitation. Joint statement in association with the resuscitation council*. BMA House, London: March

Bradshaw A (1996) The spiritual dimension of hospice: The secularization of an ideal. *Soc Sci Med* **43**(3): 409–19

Buckman R (1996) Talking to patients about cancer. *Br Med J* **313**: 699–700

Calman K, Hine D (1995) *A Policy Framework for Commissioning Cancer Services*. Department of Health, Welsh Office, London

Cherney NI (1998) Commentary. Sedation in response to refactory existential distress. Walking the final line. *J Pain Symptom Manage* **16**(6)

Clark D (1999) Cradled to the grave? Terminal care in the UK 1948–67. *Mortality* **4**(3): 225–247

Clover A, Kassab S (1998) Complementary medicine for patients with cancer. *Eur J Palliat Care* **5**(3): 73–76

Collins English Dictionary (1995) The Institutionalisation of the Good Death. *Soc Sci Med* **39**(11): 1501–8

Conill C *et al* (1997) Sympton prevalence in the last week of life. *J Pain Symptom Manage* **14**(6): 328–331

Corner J (1997) More openness needed in palliative care. *Br Med J* **315**: 1242

Corner J, Dunlop R (1997) New Approaches to Care. In: Clark D, Hockey J, Ahmedzai S (eds) *New Themes in Palliative Care*. Open University Press, Buckingham

Craig GM (1996) On withholding artificial hydration and nutrition from terminally ill-sedated patients. The debate continues. *J Med Ethics* 22(3): 147–153

Davis A (1996) Ethics and ethnicity: End-of-life decisions in four ethnic groups of cancer patients. *Med Law* **15**(3): 429–432

Department of Health (1998) *Palliative Care Health Service Circular HSC 1998/115*. The Department of Health, Wetherby: June

Donelly S (1999) Folklore associated with dying in the west of Ireland. *Palliat Med* **13**: 57–62

Doyle D (1998) Domicillary Palliative Care. In: Doyle D, Hanks G, MacDonald N *Oxford Textbook of Palliative Medicine*. 2nd edn. Oxford University Press, New York: 657–953

Dunlop RJ *et al* (1995) On withholding artificial hydration and nutrition in the terminally ill; Has palliative medicine gone too far? *J Med Ethics* **21**(3): 141–43

Dunphy K *et al* (1995) Rehydration in palliative and terminal care: If not why not? *Palliat Med* **9**: 221–228

Dunphy K, Randall F (1997) Ethical decision making in palliative care. *Eur J Palliat Care* **4**(4): 126–128

Ellershaw JE, Peat SJ, Boys LC (1995) Assessing the effectiveness of a hospital palliative care team. *Palliat Med* **9**(2): 145–152

Escalante CP, Martin CG, Elting LSR *et al* (1997) Medical futility and appropriate medical care in patients whose death is thought to be imminent. *Support Care Cancer* **5**(4): 274–80

Eve A, Smith AM, Tebbit P (1997) Hospice and palliative care trends in the uk 1994–5, including a summary of trends 1990–5. *Palliat Med* **11**: 31–43

Farsides CCS (1998) Autonomy and its implications for palliative care: a northern european perspective. *Palliat Med* **12**: 147–151

Feuer D (1998) Organ donation in palliative care. *Eur J Palliat Care* **5**(1): 21–25

Field D (1994) Palliative medicine and the medicalization of death. *Eur J Cancer Care* **3**: 58–62

Fordham S, Dowrick C, May C (1998) Palliative medicine: Is it really specialist territory? *J Royal Soc Med* **91**: 568–572

Gannon C (1995) Letter. *Br J Gen Prac* **45**(400): 630

Garwin M (1998) The duty to care – the right to refuse. *J Legal Med* **19**: 99–125

Gaze MN *et al* (1997) Pain relief and quality of life following radiotherapy for bone metastases; a randomised trial of two fractionation schedules. *Radiother Oncol* **45**: 109–116

Grande GE, Barclay SIG, Todd CJ (1997) Difficulty of symptom control and general practitoners knowledge of patients' symptoms. *Palliat Med* **11**: 399–406

Griffiths A, Beaver K (1997) Quality of life during high dose chemotherapy for breast cancer. *Int J Palliat Nurs* **3**(3): 138–144

Hanson LC, Danis M, Garret J (1997) Reflections on death and dying. *Acad Med* **72**(10): 848–855

Hardy J (1996) Endocrine therapy in advanced malignancy. *Eur J Palliat Care* **2**(4): 151–154

Higginson IJ (1998) Who needs palliative care? *J Royal Soc Med* **91**(11): 563–564

Higginson IJ, Astin P, Dolan S (1998) Where do cancer patients die? Ten year trends in the place of death of cancer patients in England. *Palliat Med* **12**: 353–363

Hinton J (1994) Which patients with terminal cancer are admitted from home care? *Palliat Med* **8**: 197–210

Holstein M (1997) The naturalness of dying. *JAMA* **273**(13): 1039–43

Hunt R (1997) Place of death of cancer patients; choice versus constraint. *Prog Palliat Care* **5**(6): 238–242

Illich I (1990) *Limits to Medicine, Medical Nemesis: the expropriation of health*. Penguin Ltd, London

Jeffery P, Millard PH (1997) An ethical framework for clinical Decision-making at the end of life. *J Royal Soc Med* **90**: 504–506

Johnson IS, Rogers C, Biswas B, Ahmedzai S (1990) What do hospices do? *Br Med J* **300**: 791–793

Joint Working Party of the National Council for Hospices and Specialist Palliative Care Services and the Association for Palliative Medicine of Great Britain and Ireland (1997) CPR for people who are terminally ill. *Eur J Palliat Care* **4**(4): 125

Joint Working Party of the National Council for Hospices and Specialist Palliative Care Services and the Association for Palliative Medicine of Great Britain and Ireland (1997) Artificial hydration (AH) for people who are terminally ill. *Eur J Palliat Care* **4**(4): 126–128

Kite SM *et al* (1998) Development of an aromatherapy service at a cancer centre. *Palliat Med* **12**: 171–180

Latimer E (1991) Caring for seriously ill and dying patients: the philosophy and ethics. *CMAJ* **144**(7): 859–864

Maddocks I (1998) Explaining palliative care — to the law and to others. *Prog Palliat Care* **6**(3): 67–68

Maiwand MO (1998) Cryotherapy for management of endobronchial obstruction. *CME Bulletin Palliative Medicine* **1**(1): Aug/Sept

Mason JK, McCall, Smith RA (1991) *Law and Medical Ethics.* 3rd edn. Butterworth, London

McCaffrey-Boyle D (1998) The cultural context of dying from cancer. *Int J Palliat Nurs* **4**(2): 70–83

McCue JD (1994) Adult Refusal of Treatment. *WLR* **290**

McNamara B, Waddell C, Colvin M (1995) Threats to the Good Death: the cultural context of stress and coping among hospice nurses. *Sociology of Health and Illness* **17**(2): 222–244

McNamara B, Waddell C, Colvin M (1994) The institutionalisation of the 'good death'. *Soc Sci Med* **39**(11): 1501–8

Meystre CJN, Burley NMJ, Ahmedzai S (1997) What investigations and procedures do patients in hospices want? Inverview based survey on patients and their nurses. *Br Med J* **315**: 1202–03

Middleton GW *et al* (1998) Good symptom relief with palliative MVP (Mitomycin-C Vinglastine and Cisplatin) chemotherapy in malignant mesothelioma. *Ann Oncol* **9**: 269–273

Moe C, Schroll M (1998) Choice of treatment among residents of nursing homes in case of life threatening Disease (English summary). *Ugeskr Laeger* **26:160**(5): 638–643

Morrison RS, Morris J (1995) When there is no cure: Palliative care for the dying patient. *Geriatrics* **50**(7): 45–51

National Council for Hospice and Specialist Palliative Services (1995) *Occasional Paper 8 Specialist Palliative Care: A Statement of Definitions.* National Council for Hospice and Specialist Palliative Services, London: Oct

National Council for Hospice and Specialist Paliative Services (1998) *A Guide to the Commissioning of Palliative Care Services for Adults.* National Council for Hospice and Specialist Palliative Services, London

National Council for Hospice and Specialist Palliative Services (1997) *Voluntary Euthanasia: The Council's View.* National Council for Hospice and Specialist Palliative Services, London: July

NHS Executive (1995) Cover for the Expert Advisory Group on Cancer to the Medical Officer for England and Wales. *A Policy Framework for Commissioning Cancer Services*. EL 95(5) April. NHS Executive, London: April

NHS Executive (1996) *A Policy Framework for Commissioning Cancer Services: Palliative Care Services*. EL 960 85: NHS Executive, London: ref 58

NHS Executive (1996) *Executive Letter (EL) (96085)*. The NHS Executive, London: ref 42

Nyatanga L (1998) Professional ethnocentricism and shared learning. Guest editorial, *Nurse Ed Today* **18**(3): 175–177

Palmer C, Higginson I, Jones P (1998) Hospice at home (letter). *Br J Gen Pract* **1006**: Feb

Payne SA, Langley-Evans A, Hillier R (1996) Perceptions of a Good Death: Comparative study of the views of hospice staff and patients. *Palliat Med* **10**: 307–312

Re C (1998) Commentary: Sedation in response to refractory existential distress: walking the fine line. *J Pain Symptom Manage* **16**(6): 404–405

Rogue D, Temon N, Albarede J *et al* (1994) Questions raised by artificial prolongation of life in the aged patient. *Med Law* **13**: 269–375

St Christoper's Hospice Information Service (1998) *Directory of Hospice and Palliative Care Services in the United Kingdom and Ireland*. Hospice Information Service, St Christopher's Hospice, London

Saunders C (1998) Caring for cancer. *J Royal Soc Med* **91**: 439–441

Saunders C (1994) Letter. *Eur J Cancer Care*: 148

Seale C, Addington-Hall J, McCarthy M (1997) Awareness of dying: prevalence, causes and consequences. *Soc Sci Med* **45**(3): 477–84

Seamark DA, Thorne CP, Lawrence C, Gray DJ (1995) Appropriate place of death for cancer patients; views of general practitioners and hospital doctors. *Br J Gen Pract* **45**(396): 359–63

Shaiova L (1998) Case Presentation: Terminal sedation and existential distress. *J Pain Symptom Manage* **16**(6): 403–404

Silvestri G, Pritchard R, Welch HG (1998) Preferences for chemotherapy in patients with advanced non-small cell lung cancer: Descriptive study based on scripted interviews. *Br Med J* **317**: 771–775

Slevin M *et al* (1990) Attitudes to chemotherapy: comparing views of patients with cancer with those of doctors, nurses and general public. *Br Med J* **300**: 1458–60

Stanley JM (1992) The Appleton International Conference:
Developing Guidelines for Decisions to Forego Life-
Prolonging Medical Treatment. *J Med Ethics* **18**(suppl): 3–5

Swanson JW, McCrary SV (1996) Medical futility decisions and
physicians' legal defensiveness: the impact of anticipated
conflicts on thresholds for end-of-life treatment. *Soc Sci Med*
42(1): 125–132

Thatcher N, Anderson H, Betticher DC *et al* (1995) Symptomatic
benefit from gencitabine and other chemotherapy in
advanced non-small cell lung cancer: Changes in performance
status and tumour related symptoms. *Anti-cancer drugs* **6**(6):
39–48

The Editor (1998) Change and progress (editorial). *Progr Palliat
Care* **6**(1): 1–3

The Expert Advisory Group on Cancer (1995) *A Policy
Framework for Commissioning Cancer Services*. The
Department of Health and the Welsh Office, March

Thorns A (1998) A review of the Doctrine of Double Effect. *Eur J
Palliat Care* **5**(4): 117–120

Thorns A (1998) Doctrine of double effect means that death is
not intended (letter). *Br Med J* **316**(31): January

Tong KL, Spicer BJ (1994) The chinese palliative patient and
family in north america: A cultural perspective. *J Palliat
Care* **10**(1): 26–28

Twycross R (1997) *Symptom Management in Advanced Cancer*.
2nd edn. Radcliffe Medical Press, Oxford

Vainio A, Auvinen A with Members of the Symptom Prevalence
Group (1996) Prevalence of symptoms among patients with
advanced cancer: an international collaborative study. *J Pain
Symptom Manage* **12**(1): 3–10

World Health Organization (1990) *Cancer Pain Relief and
Palliative Care: report of a WHO Expert Committee*. WHO,
Geneva

World Health Organization (1958) *The First Ten Years. The
Health Organization*. WHO, Geneva

5

Ethical issues surrounding death and dying

Simon Chippendale

For Emma and Charles,

*May your lives find increasing value,
be valuable and be valued by others.*

The previous chapter considered some of the challenges healthcare professionals' face in providing palliative care that is appropriate, of high quality and yet remains meaningful to the dying person, their family and their carers. Professionals involved in such care are increasingly faced with ethical dilemmas as they seek to fulfil their respective caring goals. On the one hand, quality is directly influenced by the changing circumstances of healthcare provision which when combined with current advances and developments in healthcare treatments adds increasing financial burden on currently limited budgets. On the other hand, quality can be determined subjectively by the perspectives of the patient, their carers and their family. Those responsible for the provision of palliative care should be aware of what would be ideal; equally they are responsible for managing their budgets in a realistic manner and with finite resources.

This chapter considers the current influences on ethics in our society, which help to explain the moral picture against which ethical decisions are made. Two key theories to determine whether the moral picture is ethically permissible are consequentialism and deontology. Other theories could be considered, but for the sake of brevity and the more common approach to healthcare, the justification of the moral argument has been restricted to these two approaches. In determining the ethical permissibility of clinical situations four key principles for healthcare ethics are introduced, ie. the principle of respect for autonomy, beneficience, non-maleficience and justice. Examples are given to illustrate the potential for conflict.

The temptation in determining what is ethically permissible is to consider the values held by the healthcare professionals in the situation who, while not deliberately ignoring the needs of the patient and their families, are failing to take the time to explore and consider the ethical implications of actions with them. Death is the one common denominator among all humans, Simone de Beauvoir (1969) recalled a comment made by her dying mother, 'Death does not frighten me; it is the jump I am afraid of'. The ethics involved need not focus on the morals of death but on the manner in which death is attained, the ethics behind the 'jump'.

When making decisions ethicists justify their decisions or argue their position and the validity of their reasoning focusing on the overall moral picture and the ethical permissibility of their actions within the moral picture. Frequently the moral picture becomes complicated; the skill in ensuring care is ethically permissible lies in determining what the actual moral picture being debated really is. Conflict can arise in the ethical acceptability of the situation and subsequently in the desirability of some situations. One theoretical approach, deontology, utilises a tool called the *doctrine of double effect* (mentioned briefly in *Chapter 4*) that permits deontologists to find some actions ethically permissible despite certain foreseeable consequences that would not normally be justifiable for deontologists. The *acts and omissions* doctrine argues that under normal circumstances it is ethically more preferable to accept less favourable results of actions from omissions of care, than to accept equivalent results from a deliberate action. There is contention that there remains no difference between actions or omissions of care, that there is no ethical difference in the intention to act or to omit care (Rachels, 1975). This has particular relevance to the withholding and withdrawal of treatments, especially near the end of life. These latter two concepts will be outlined and applied to clinical examples to illustrate further potential for conflict and resolution within palliative healthcare provision.

Palliative care can lead to the greatest challenge, especially in determining the ethical aspects of dying and of death. Healthcare professionals are aware of what they want to provide to maximise a person's quality of life, particularly where a person is dying. The focus of care is on improving the quality of life for the person and their family in a manner that is acceptable and wanted by the patient. Conflict might occur when the patient (perhaps in conjunction with their family) feels that they have reached a point where their perception of their quality of life is so poor that, in some circumstances, death becomes a preferable option. Ending suffering is seen as more desirable than allowing it to continue, despite the efforts of healthcare professionals to alleviate the suffering.

The ethical permissibility in this area focuses on the quality of life versus the sanctity of life. Currently in English law there is a prohibition on the killing or deliberate taking of a human life. The professional bodies for healthcare professionals reflect this deontological sentiment placing emphasis on a duty of care and not harming a patient. This works for deontological style ethicists, but for those of consequential persuasion there is a balance between the quality of life (making a life worthwhile) and its duration and the extent of imposed 'suffering' compared with the implication of hastening the end of that life. Both notions require an ethical justification of the value of life based on ethical principles.

The ethics surrounding palliative care are frequently dominated by the debate surrounding euthanasia, which is a worthwhile debate in itself and focuses on both the sanctity and value of life. By its definition, palliative care neither hastens nor prolongs death (Twycross, 1999). This is supported by the National Council for Hospice and Specialist Palliative Care Services (NCHSPCS), (1997) guidelines regarding voluntary euthanasia. This places emphasis on improving the remaining quality of life for the dying person,

> *... the intention of good palliative care for dying patients is to relieve their physical, emotional, social and spiritual suffering in the context of respect for their individuality, and without the intent to shorten life.*
>
> (NCHSPCS, 1997)

Subsequently in palliative care there can be little consideration for euthanasia apart from recognising the potential influence that it exerts on the provision of high quality care. Euthanasia suggests the ending of life by passive or active means, in the voluntary or non-voluntary capacities of the dying person. It suggests a premature ending of life which is in conflict with the ethos of palliative care. The only potential for consideration within palliative care could be where caring professionals respect the autonomous wishes of a dying person not to commence further treatments but to continue to provide the basic care required. This omission of 'care' is perhaps as close to passive, voluntary euthanasia that palliative care could ever get.

This chapter invites the reader to reflect on the issues surrounding the ethics involved and, where appropriate, to discuss them with a colleague or to read further.

The moral picture

This is the framework in which individuals or groups of people interact, where their actions or inactions have a direct effect on others. In ethics, the moral picture requires the individual to put aside emotive feelings about the subject and to engage in an objective discussion about the issues involved, depending on their particular philosophical school of thought. To illustrate the differences between consequentialist and deontological thinking the following simplified moral picture should be considered,

A can do X to B with the result being Y

Consequentialist approaches

Consequentialists consider the prime consideration in determining whether something is ethically permissible or not is to look at the consequences in the moral picture. The ethical permissibility of the action (or inaction) X, is determined on the acceptability of the consequences Y. For hedonistic consequentialists the goal for acceptable consequences are those that maximise 'happiness' or benefit, and minimise harm. There are other styles of consequentialism or utilitarianism, act- and rule-utilitarians. Act-utilitarians consider the consequences for each individual moral picture, while rule-based utilitarians consider the moral picture, determine what is ethically permissible and apply this to all similar situations.

Difficulties arise for consequentialists in determining the overall benefit, as some actions lead to both good and bad effects, the benefit being seen only from the perspective of those wishing the actions to be ethically permitted. Additional difficulty arises in determining the amount of benefit or minimum sadness; what if action X could be spread to many but be diluted to give a little happiness to a greater number. How might this compare with giving action X to a single person where it could provide the maximum benefit, but only for that one person? Whose is the greater need? While both are good, is one of greater ethical permissibility? A final issue for consequentialist determination depends on whether an individual or group decide that their pleasure or happiness can only be obtained through X which would be considered by others not to be a pleasure or happiness, or that their pleasure X is derived from a harm instigated on others.

Deontological approaches

Deontologists live according to categorical imperatives; simply stated these are a set of rules or guidelines that govern their actions, for example, not killing or telling lies. The ethical permissibility of the moral picture focuses on the action X for which you are responsible. As long as X is ethically permissible then it is of no significance what the consequences Y become. The difficulty here is that by adhering to some ethical principles as a deontologist can have disastrous consequences for others involved in the moral picture. Where certain actions which are desirable in the moral picture might result in foreseeable consequences that are harmful, the deontologist would refer to a tool known as the *Doctrine of Double Effect* (DDE) to determine whether the action was ethically permissible. This tool is often misquoted by the media, it could never make killing ethically acceptable for deontologists.

Campbell and Collinson (1988) offer an appropriate summary of the DDE,

> *The Doctrine of Double Effect says that, in certain conditions, you need not be responsible for those effects of your actions which, though foreseen, are not intended.*

In other words, it can make some actions that might have certain foreseeable side-effects ethically permissible provided that four conditions are met. These are,

1. 'What is done must be, at the least, morally permissible.
2. What is intended must include only the good and not the bad effects of what is done.
3. The bad effects must not be the means whereby the good is brought about.
4. There must be proportionality between the good and the bad effects of what is done.'

(Campbell and Collinson, 1988: 155)

This becomes significant for deontologists within palliative care since this would ethically permit an action that would relieve suffering, although a possible side-effect caused further harm to the patient.

Question

> * *How might a situation occur in palliative care where deontologists use the DDE to ethically justify specific treatments, or the withdrawal of care?*

The result of these two simplified outlines of consequentialism and deontology is that the differing approaches can both find ethically permissible actions or inactions that may be in conflict, particularly in the clinical situation. Healthcare professionals work within codes of conduct that govern their approaches to care. These generally require a duty of care to the patient. Subsequently, health professional's work can be greatly influenced from deontological perspectives. While the healthcare professional might perceive from the holistic nature of their palliative care that alternative consequences might be more desirable they can find that their care is governed and regulated by responsibilities and duties for which they become accountable.

An example of conflict that can arise between deontologists and consequentialists can be illustrated by the following:

A person enters an enclosed room where you are gathered with a large group of your colleagues and friends. She has a weapon, she indicates that you have a choice, either you can end the lives of three members of the group, or she will end the lives of everyone in the room leaving you until last.

Questions

* *What would you do in such a situation?*
* *Would your decisions change if the group of people changed, eg. colleagues, strangers, close family, children, old people, patients, people who had been diagnosed with an incurable disease?*
* *How might your actions change and differ in your professional capacity? What influenced the change and why?*

A consequential approach may be to recognise that while the deaths of three members of the group is harmful, this is offset by the saving of the lives of all the others in the group. The overall consequences are more beneficial than if everyone is killed; subsequently for a consequentialist the decision to go along with the killing of three members of the group can be considered to be ethically permissible (to the relief of those who survive).

Should you hold stronger deontological views, then you recognise that killing is not ethically permissible. Subsequently you are forced to choose the latter option offered by the terrorist. This results in the deaths of the entire group — but the decision that you made was ethically justifiable. The responsibility for the action of killing and for the deaths of the group remained with the person brandishing the gun.

This example illustrates how differing approaches to ethics can result in potential conflict: where one approach finds certain actions or inactions which have a harmful result to be ethically permissible, another approach would never consider such actions or inaction's.

Principles of healthcare ethics

In determining whether the subject has received benefit or harm there are four key ethical principles that need to be considered. Identified by Beauchamp and Childress (1994) as the principles of respect, autonomy, beneficience, non-maleficience and justice, these principles form the ethical building blocks from which individual circumstances can be considered.

The principle of respect for autonomy

This is perhaps the strongest consideration in making clinical decisions. Respecting the autonomy of another requires that person to be actively involved in the decision-making process. Without such consultation, any decisions made on their behalf and for their benefit would be tantamount to paternalism. This is of particular relevance to dying people because they can develop conditions or have decreased levels of consciousness where they are unable to be consulted and/or to make informed knowledgeable decisions for themselves. In the absence of family members or friends who are able to make decisions for that person, clinical decisions are left for the multi-professional team to determine. Their guide in making such decisions shall be to ensure that all decisions taken are in the best interests of the patient.

Gillon (1986) defines autonomy as,

> ... the capacity to think, decide, and act on the basis of such thought and decision freely and independently and without... let or hindrance.

(Gillon, 1986: 60)

Gillon further suggests that the key components to autonomy include, the ability to think, the freedom of will to be able to do things that one wants, and finally, to be able to perform one's desired wishes.

Questions

* *How might the autonomy of a person who is dying be compromised?*
* *When might the paternalistic behaviour of healthcare professionals at the end of life, be justified?*
* *How could the respect of the dying patient's autonomy be maximised in such circumstances?*

As a person, you might have very strong preferences about how you might die and where. It is likely that you would consider these points to be very important, and while you are able to discuss and 'protect' your interests, your autonomy is likely to be respected. Unfortunately there are circumstances where, through illness and disease, the person who is dying is less able to 'protect' their individual autonomy and becomes increasingly vulnerable. This can be the result of:

* either the spread of the disease or illness and its effects on how people communicate their needs
* being physically unable to respond
* being unable to understand the information and make decisions based upon the information.

Also, mind-altering chemicals can compromise autonomy, such as alcohol or certain medication.

Autonomy may also be compromised by having the ability to choose one's circumstances removed or through coercion, or even the non-provision of sufficient information on which to make a choice. Autonomy is strongly related to consent; where autonomy is respected then healthcare professionals are required to obtain consent for actions or procedures performed.

As people who are dying become increasingly unconscious, their ability to maintain their autonomy can be diminished. In the absence of a recent living will, families should be consulted as to what might be in the best interests of the patient; in the absence of close family or of a person appointed by the dying patient then healthcare professionals are forced to act in paternalistic manners. This encroaches on the autonomy of the patient while maintaining that no harm is done to the patient.

Beneficience and non-maleficience

At their simplest these principles are to do good and to do no harm respectively. There is some debate over which should take precedence although it would seem more appropriate for the latter to have priority. A dying person who was unable to communicate a preference would clearly benefit from having less harm inflicted on them rather than a transitory favourable moment.

Beneficience is tempered by the principle of respect for autonomy of the patient, in that this is what he really wants. It is also tempered by non-maleficience, ie. the benefit offered to one might cause harm to others by depriving them of a similar opportunity? Equally, beneficience is tempered by the principle of justice; harm may be perpetuated if the 'benefit' is not available to all. Healthcare professionals have autonomy and a right for their professional autonomy to be respected. They should not therefore be expected to perform actions that challenge the fairness of distribution.

Questions

* *What makes a 'good moment', good or preferable?*
* *What makes a 'bad moment' bad or harmful?*
* *What influences our decisions in our everyday lives?*
* *How might beneficience and non-maleficience influence factors at the end of life?*

Non-maleficience in the care of the dying person can appear to be a desirable principle, however there is a balance between harm induced and its potential benefit. Individuals are normally happy to accept the sharp intra-muscular injections of analgesia for long-term pain relief. In palliative care, treatment that is considered ordinary at an early stage in a patient's disease might be seen as extraordinary treatment near the end of life. The adverse side-effects of chemotherapy are tolerated when there is hope of a beneficial cure for the disease. There are circumstances where a dying person might elect to undergo a short term harm-inducing procedure because this is outweighed by the long term benefit resulting from this procedure. Equally, the difficulty of ensuring beneficience by declining treatments which can prevent further suffering could become of prime importance. This relates to the acts and omission doctrine, where Rachels's argues (1975) that both have equal weight in their moral outcome; there is no moral difference between an action or an omission. It also relates to whether treatments can be considered to be ordinary or extraordinary.

Justice

In ethics justice is not the retributive style of justice, but ensures fairness and equality. This is difficult to maintain in a society and culture full of social inequalities. However the principle of equality for all remains. In coming to ethical decisions the question of actions or omissions needs considering: any action or omission of care provided for one person should be available for all. For those who are dying, this suggests that whatever is done to care for one person should be provided for all other similar patients, and that there can be no place for the rationing of healthcare based on illness and disease, age or infirmity.

Questions

* *What are the resources that you control on a daily basis in your professional capacity?*
* *How do you decide how to distribute these resources?*
* *How do you ensure equality and equity in your distribution?*

Paternalism

Paternalism is making decisions on behalf of others in their best interests. Although intrinsically beneficial, paternalistic actions might not respect the individual autonomy of that person or group or their ability to choose for themselves given the appropriate information. A harmful action cannot be considered to be paternalistic, it remains harmful. Paternalism might not be considered to be ethically justifiable within a deontological system. It could be considered to harm the rights of the person or group and therefore could not form the basis of a universal law. Consequentialists would consider the overall benefit to be derived from the situation and may find paternalistic action, in some instances, ethically permissible. In healthcare paternalism has been accepted where patients are unable to make decisions for themselves, particularly in situations where a person's 'competence' is diminished. This tends to reflect a consequential approach to decision-making and frequently occurs within palliative care with the onset of unconsciousness, or of a person becoming increasingly unable to take decisions for themselves due to diseases affecting their ability to make rational decisions.

It could be argued that where a person's autonomy is diminished by circumstances, paternalism becomes increasingly justifiable, particularly where no other person has been appointed to act as a proxy consent. At times, though decisions are made on the patient's behalf citing that the person could not understand the information required, the issue is whether the person has actually been consulted, offered the choice of whether they wish to know, or even if the information has been simplified while retaining accuracy in order for them to understand better and come to their own decision. Time is a large factor in such situations, but needs to be made available, particularly within palliative care.

Questions

* *Could paternalism be used to justify withdrawal of care in the end of life situations?*
* *What steps could be taken to try to minimise paternalistic actions at the end of life?*
* *To what extent are you aware of paternalistic action being adopted within your area of work? (Does this extend to meal times, taking vital signs etc.?)*

Clinical decisions

As with all aspects of healthcare, respecting the autonomy of the individual is of paramount ethical importance in palliative care. This can be achieved by at least attempting to maximise the opportunity for the patient to receive information, to understand, to come to a personal decision and to communicate that decision freely. In clinical situations this is not always possible. Difficulties may result from either the competence of the patient being diminished or through the paternalistic behaviour of healthcare providers. Even where the patient is competent and fulfills the abilities described above, he or she can come to a decision that the quality of his/her life is minimal, and that his/her personal condition maximises suffering. In such instances it is understandable why an individual might decide that he would prefer his life to end. This is a very individual decision, by no means an easy one to come to, and is best made in consultation with close family in order that they can understand the patient's reasoning. Ultimately, this must represent a failure of care, physical, psychological, emotional, social and spiritual in attempting to maximise the quality of life for the patient, to enable them to live until they die. Such decisions challenge the ethics of healthcare in that carers are unable to provide what the patient requires. Healthcare professionals could not act on a declaration of wanting life to end, even when made by a fully autonomous person. They are bound by their professional codes of conduct, not to harm (the ending of a life) patients. This may not be as clear-cut for healthcare professionals as they might like particularly when they hold personal consequentialist views. A carer may see the continued and prolonged suffering endured by the dying patient and family as harmful in situations where adequate palliative care is not provided or is insufficient to maintain the quality of life for the patient who is dying.

In some instances the health service is keeping people alive longer than their physical bodies can hope to repair. There is a recognisable difference between stopping the working of a ventilator following criteria for brain stem death being satisfied and withholding food where a person has a diagnosis of being in persistent vegetative state. Here, the equivalent ending of life (even with the agreement of family) could be considered harmful in that withholding food would be an omission of care; a withdrawal of the means by which the patient was fed would be an action (eg. removal of a feeding tube), ensuring a slower death. Is there a moral difference between the action of switching off a ventilator and the removal of a feeding tube? In one case, parts of the brain are able to function unaided; in the other, the parts of the brain essential to maintain life are irrecoverably damaged. There is a difference in comparing the category of patient. It would appear that where the body's vital signs are naturally maintained then this is of sufficient interest to warrant closer attention and consideration of whether that life can be ethically ended by deliberate action. The situation needs to determine whether the care of the dying person is ordinary or extraordinary, and where the boundary from being ordinary to extraordinary treatments for dying people crosses.

Questions

* *What constitutes ordinary care and extra-ordinary care for a person who is dying?*
* *Who is likely to determine this?*
* *When and how might ordinary care become extraordinary care at the end of life?*
* *What determines how far extraordinary care is offered to dying people?*
* *How might this influence the quality of their life, and of their dying?*
* *If the extraordinary care can't be offered to every person who wants it, should it be offered at all?*

Death and dying

In considering the ethics surrounding death and dying the question of whether a difference exists between the two states needs to be addressed. Should greater value be placed on life? Death is the unknown factor, an event which people are aware of but know nothing.

> *Human death is an unknown, surrounded by myth, dreams, fears, uncertainties and distress of all kinds.*

> (Campbell *et al*, 1997)

Death is a distinct event that every human will encounter, a certainty that might not respect individual autonomous wishes. Can death have ethical considerations? If value is placed on living then there should be equal value on the manner of dying or on the ending of life. If life should be respected, then it would be appropriate to respect the manner of dying. While death is a certainty, there is no choice about it. It is the vulnerability of individuals who are dying that needs to be recognised. It is for this reason that healthcare workers should consider the ethical basis of their care and how decisions about that care are reached in order not to take advantage of the vulnerable person.

Death can be both beneficial and non-maleficient, particularly where it offers a release from suffering. Above all, it is perhaps the most accurate and appropriately distributed notion of justice that could be considered, it comes to everyone.

Perhaps it is not death that has strong ethical connections but the manner in which death comes that has the greater ethical significance. Neuberger (1999) places emphasis on recognising the spiritual aspects of dying within care provided. She encourages a societal change to the subject of death and dying to make the face of death more acceptable and less frightening.

> *We will only achieve a real change, allowing ourselves to express our fears and hopes and desires if we are able and prepared to face the issue of how best to meet our end, and the end of others we love and respect, by discussing, talking, arguing, planning, and by resolving to improve what is still a very patchy situation in this country, where we only get the chance of having a good death by battling against the odds.*

(Neuberger, 1999)

Death can be the result of natural old age, disease, natural accidents and disasters, we consider these deaths 'acts of God' and are perhaps relieved that we were not in that part of creation to experience the phenomenon, but are duly reminded of our frail mortality. Death can arrive through accidents and unforeseeable consequences are seen as being unfortunate and untimely. Under these circumstances death is neutral, the ending of life through natural and unplanned action. Death can also be brought about by deliberate circumstance, killing through war, suicide, sacrifice, murder, euthanasia and capital punishment. Is there a difference between the ethical notions of the manner in which death is brought about?

The issue of what is morally wrong with death can be considered. Glover (1977) would suggest that there is little wrong with death, only in killing. Killing is not wrong in that it deprives a person of his/her intrinsic value of life, but because killing reduces the length of a 'worthwhile' life. The killing of a person who would want to go on living or killing in a manner that causes fear or harm prior to the death is wrong. Killing is also wrong due to the harmful effect on those left behind, and the deprivation of the dead person's contribution to society. In the same way that killing can be seen as morally bad, the saving of life becomes increasingly morally acceptable, making it harder to justify ethically the hastening of death whatever the circumstances.

Questions

* *What makes life and living 'worthwhile'?*
* *How might you determine at what point a life is considered to be no longer 'worthwhile' at the end of life?*

The notion of killing has differing degrees of acceptability, the killing of a child or elderly person unable to defend themselves is considered worse than that of a person who could defend him/herself. Until 1961, the killing of self was considered to be an illegal act. In contrast, self-killing could be considered to be more valuable in the sacrificial sense where the lives of others are saved, eg. the fighter pilot who does not eject from a stricken plane in order to ensure it does not crash into a village, or a person who saves the life of another but in doing so recognises that he is putting his own life at great risk. The manner of these deaths appears to be ethically preferable to others, in that the death gains value. There remains the ethical question of whether the manner of this death is ethically acceptable, or as ethically acceptable as suicide. If this is more ethically acceptable then how should the views of a mother or father wishing to donate their heart (given it to be perfect match) for their only child be considered?

The difference between these manners of killing becomes one of how benefit is measured, and whether there is proportionality between the two sets of circumstances. The consequences become valuable in determining the ethical permissibility. While accepted by consequentialists, deonto-logists use the DDE to find such actions ethically permissible. Misplaced media misinformation can often determine whether the manner of death is morally acceptable in the eyes of society. The manner of dying can appear on the surface to be more acceptable in some guises.

The taking of a life is morally wrong. It deprives the person of his/her life, it deprives others of the person's continued contribution to their lives and it does not respect the autonomy of the person if they do not wish to die at that moment.

There are circumstances where a patient chooses to die, to retain their right to choose to end their life. Where competent, this is an autonomous choice and can be respected as a decision. The NCHSPCS (1997) recognised the right of the individual to wish to die; however, the challenge for healthcare professionals occurs where the wish becomes a request to assist in the hastening of death for a patient. This situation remains illegal within English law. It crosses the divide of what is ethically permissible, particularly for deontologists. While we need to respect the autonomy of others, which can include their wish to die, this has to be tempered with their respect of our own autonomy of not wishing to kill a person.

While the moral wrongness of **killing** is recognised by Glover (1977), who offers a sound argument as to why it is ethically wrong to take a life, another ethical consideration is what **value** has life. If life has value then it becomes unethical to deprive a person of it. Harris (1985) considers that what makes life valuable is not based on equity across all people but the capacity to value our lives as well as that of others. Subsequently the inherent wrong in killing is to deprive a person of the capacity to value their lives. While this argument supports the notion that the killing of a life is wrong in itself, there is another consideration. Where a person does not value his life, can depriving him of life be considered to be morally wrong? It is perhaps then that it is the manner of dying that becomes important. The issue of Harris's capacity for life also becomes important in consideration of dying: does a person have the capacity to appreciate the manner in which they are dying, if they do not have that capacity then would it be ethically acceptable to deprive them of their life by killing them?

While capacity to value is appropriate for those who are competent to determine and articulate what they want, there is an issue for those whose personal autonomy is restricted, for example, if unconscious. Living wills enable the wishes of the person to be stated at a point in time when the living will is written. While not indicating current wishes and although not legally binding, the living will can provide insight into the feelings and wishes of dying patients, indicating their preferences. They should not include directions to actually end the life of the person; this could not be ethically permitted and should be ignored by carers.

Concluding thoughts

The sanctity of life would appear to mirror the value of life, and where there is value of life it should not be prematurely ended. The ethics of dying and death need to consider the individual manner of dying and the person's fears, concerns and other wishes. It would be ethically preferable to work to maintain the dying person's quality of life, while recognising the individual nature of death and the circumstances surrounding dying and death. Careful consideration of the ethics involved in differing situations enable ethically based permissible care to be provided. Dame Cecily Saunders comments on the importance of caring for those who are dying, recognising that what becomes important is enabling someone to live until they die. Appropriate consideration of ethical principles, together with recognition of how they are being applied can enable carers to provide ethically justifiable actions or omissions that enable the patient to live their life more fully to the point where they die.

Randall and Downie (1999) in discussion about the value of life conclude that,

Values are in the end personal preferences, but ethics is a system of interpersonal rules for the better ordering of human life.

(p.304)

In determining the ethics of dying, careful consideration of ethical rules, recognition of where they have come from and their influences on our personal lives, should ensure that the care offered to those who are dying and their families is not just justifiable and permissible, but appropriate for that person while remaining within professional boundaries.

The principles of healthcare ethics provide the building blocks on which the moral picture can be explored, ethical theory provides the framework in determining the acceptability (or not) of decisions and care, be it action or omission. Carers need to utilise ethics to protect the vulnerable dying person, and to maximise the benefits in maintaining the person's quality of life.

References

Beauchamp TL, Childress JF (1994) *Principles of Biomedical Ethics*. 4th edn. Oxford University Press, Oxford

Campbell A, Charlesworth M, Gillett G *et al* (1997) *Medical Ethics*. 2nd edn. Oxford University Press, Oxford

Campbell R, Collinson D (1988) *Ending Lives*. Blackwell Publishers, Oxford

De Beauvoir S (1969) *A Very Easy Death*. Penguin Books Ltd, London

Gillon R (1986) *Philosophical Medical Ethics*. John Wiley & Sons, Chichester

Glover J (1977) *Causing Death & Saving Lives*. Penguin Ltd, London

Harris J (1985) *The Value of Life: an introduction to medical ethics*. Routledge, London

The National Council for Hospice and Specialist Palliative Care Services (1997) *Voluntary Euthanasia: The Council's View*. NCHSPCS, London

Neuberger J (1999) *Dying Well; a guide to enabling a good death.* Hochland & Hochland, Hale

Randall F, Downie R (1999) *Palliative Care Ethics; a companion for all specialities.* 2nd edn. Oxford University Press, Oxford

Rachels J (1975) Active & Passive Euthanasia. *N Engl J Med* **292**:78–80 cited by Gillon R (1986) *Philosophical Medical Ethics.* John Wiley & Sons, Chichester

Twycross R (1999) *Introducing Palliative Care.* 3rd edn. Radcliffe Medical Press, Abingdon

6

Understanding and caring for the dying patient

Brian Nyatanga

*Dying is a very dull, dreary affair. My advice to you
is to have nothing whatsoever to do with it.*

Somerset Maugham

Dying is an individual activity and therefore any care that is
going to reflect this individuality must see the patient as
central. The patient's needs (physical or psycho-emotional)
should form the basis on which the delivery and pacing of
care is determined. Such care is arguably based on a sound
understanding of the patient and family. This is important
because, although the caring professionals may become
familiar with death and dying, for the patient, death is a
unique experience, which has to be negotiated individually.
The other people around the patient can be supportive and
sensitive, and this will only help that patient with his or her
inner strength in dealing with the final encounter with
death. Caring for the dying patient must be seen as also
caring for the sum total of that patient's relations
(Nyatanga, 1993) including their multitude of emotions.
This means seeing the patient as part of a family unit. This
unit may include relatives, friends, pets and anyone the
patient considers significant, hence the term 'significant
others'.

There is a tendency to view the patient with a terminal
illness as dying and forget the positive aspect, that the same
patient is in fact still alive until he is dead. What we should
concentrate on is how to help the patient make the most (if
he/she so wishes) in terms of quality of the remaining days,
weeks or months of his life. Admittedly, palliative care is
about quality not quantity of life. A multidisciplinary team
approach to such care is a pre-requisite for palliative care to
succeed given the complex needs (physical as well as
psychological, emotional, spiritual and intellectual) presented
by the palliative patient.

Psychological dimensions of the dying

Genuine psychological care gives the patient the opportunity to analyse his own situation. This can be done by the patient asking pertinent questions, from which the answers are used to break down the matrix, in his own mind, about his illness. If this is done properly, the patient achieves more clarity of his own impending death, and this, according to Grey (1996) often leads to greater insights that permit a reintegration of self at a higher level of self-awareness and integrity. It is acknowledged that not all patients can and will ask pertinent questions but may show signs of anger or any other emotions. In this case the professionals may help the patient enter this psychological analysis by asking open-ended questions, for example, 'on top of your illness, what else is making you so angry?' The assumptions made within the question itself can be denied or nullified by the patient when he chooses his response to your open question. Admittedly, open questions allow the patient to select the most appropriate and comfortable response, enabling him/her to analyse the situation.

It can be argued that once the dying patient has accepted the reality of impending death, he/she may need to withdraw psychologically from the living world. This withdrawal is a gradual process of disengagement (Samarel, 1995) which tends to take place in the last few weeks or days of life. The patient often withdraws into himself for long periods at a time, and this may be seen as removing oneself away from the family and significant others. Disengagement is characterised by progressive lessening of verbalisation by the dying patient, increased sleep even during daytime and not wanting contact with others, including family members. It is not being suggested that disengagement takes place all the time during these last few days, but while in the process, most patients prefer not to be disturbed. It must be arduous for the patient to actively disengage from the living world that has been part of his/her life since birth. It is not the choice of the patient to disengage, but the realisation that life is soon to end in a way 'forces' him/her to engage in this process. This may not be the case with the patient who believes he still has a miraculous chance of 'beating' his illness and go on surviving. However, the actual difficulty in disengaging is that the patient has to have full concentration with minimal external distractions. In order for us the practitioners/clinicians to help the patient achieve full concentration, we need to have a fine balance when we prescribe medication that has a potential to impair such concentration while controlling other symptoms. The process of disengagement is emotionally draining for the patient and needs to be performed gradually, remaining a continuous aspect of the last few days.

During my experience of caring for dying patients in a hospice setting, I remember hearing a patient shout at her relatives to leave her alone, or in more polite terms 'not now dear'. One possible explanation for this behaviour can be attributed to the fact that the patient wanted to temporarily shut the world out and continue with disengagement. The fact that she had to shout may suggest a difference or dichotomy in perceptions between the relatives' need to spend more time with the dying patient, and the patient's need for space to disengage. According to Samarel (1995) such misunderstandings often cause distress with relatives who are not obviously aware of what is going on psychologically with the patient. The patient's need for peace and quiet must be explained to the relatives and significant others while also ensuring that the extreme opposite is avoided. The extreme opposite would be that the family, in realising this, may allow too much time apart from the patient who, in turn, may perceive this as abandonment. Samarel makes the point that the fear of abandonment is understandable, considering that dying is something that the patient does alone (*p.101*). In this case the role of the professionals would be to facilitate the achievement of a balance for the dying patient between her need for disengagement and not feeling abandoned. It does not seem an easy option at all (ie. if it is an option) to die, and hence the view being expressed in this book.

The relatives should be made aware that when a patient has peace and quiet to disengage, what he/she is basically doing is a thorough life review. A life review is about putting one's psychological and spiritual house in order. This way of introspection takes time and effort to accomplish. According to Sheldon (1997) this is a time to try and understand the painful things while remembering the successes. The patient may also want to prepare to 'travel' as a whole person (holistically) into the dying mode. This is important because in healthy life, a person's well being is very much dependent on the harmony of all the different dimensions making up that person, (ie. psychological, emotional, physical, spiritual, social and intellectual) (PEPSSI). It is therefore equally important that such harmony is ensured during dying in order to achieve a peaceful and dignified death.

Preserving self-esteem

Out of all the fears the dying patient may have, the most frightening is the loss of self-esteem. Loss of self-esteem is often seen as a violation of the very core of personal existence and individual dignity. With this violation follows the loss of control and independence. The dying patient may well understand the need for our nursing care intervention, which, at the same time, by its nature undermines his dignity and assails his sense of privacy. There does not seem to be an easier option in dying. It is well documented and acceptable that nursing care is crucial for the general comfort of the patient, as long as it is delivered in a way that does not make the patient feel less human. One example would be bowel care, which may involve giving suppositories or even performing manual evacuation. This part of care is vital, but before performing such procedures, we should ascertain the patient's previous experiences (if any) and then explain simply why the procedure is necessary. More important is the explanation of how it is going to be done. Most dying patients co-operate fully once they know the 'why' and 'how' of our care intervention.

Patients often feel that they are losing control each time the illness worsens. They may even reject what we, as professionals, perceive as sensible and helpful for them, in favour of what they believe gives them control. For example, they may struggle to the bathroom rather than use a commode by the bedside. Perhaps what professionals should constantly remind themselves is each little bit of control lost by the dying patient is a little bit of ground gained by their illness. This realisation is not easy to accept, particularly for the patient who has always been in control.

Fear of mental isolation

Apart from the observable physical isolation, the dying patient at times feels mentally isolated. There is a propensity by both relatives and professionals to jolly the patient along (Nyatanga, 1993) when he tries to express his fears and knowledge of dying. A patient may express fear of suffocating in his sleep and is afraid to sleep in case he fails to wake up. The same patient may also indicate awareness of his impending death, and wish to express his feelings. The patient may feel mentally isolated if he can not share his fears or thoughts about his dying, and is left to cope alone with his emotions. Allowing a dying patient to voice or articulate his fears often gives the family an opportunity and courage to say 'farewell' or 'I'm sorry'.

Spiritual dimension of care

Unlike psychological care which is mainly analytical in nature, spiritual care is regarded as bringing all the component parts (presumably taken apart during analysis) together, hence spiritual care is viewed as a process of synthesis (Grey 1996). The syncretistic (ability to unite) nature of spiritual care would suggest that it follows after the psychological analysis. The spiritual dimension is concerned with the essence of what it is to be human. Spirituality itself is about how individuals understand the purpose and meaning of their existence within the universe (Woof and Nyatanga, 1998). This encompasses the different aspects of a person's values, beliefs, meaning of one's existence, relationships with others and one's sense of purpose. As with relationships, Lunn (1993) suggests that these could also be with God or gods or with ourselves. Searching through the literature (Burnard, 1998; Harrison and Burnard, 1993; Smith, 1986) it seems that consideration of the spiritual is broadly based on a search for meaning. From a philosophical standpoint this is seen as a search for existential meaning in relation to a given life crisis or event. Death poses a challenge to such personally held belief systems. According to Woof and Nyatanga, some individuals possess a set of beliefs that adequately answer such a challenge, while others may end up suffering as they strive to attain inner peace.

Spiritual is often linked to or associated with religion, but these two are very different in nature (Nyatanga, 1997). It is perhaps those with a faith who may find inner peace through 'talking' to their God, Allah or Higher Power. What needs explaining is that every one of us has a spiritual dimension but may require different modalities, also known as channels, for dealing with these spiritual needs. An individual with a faith would find a religious channel the most appropriate, so involving a chaplain or head of that faith may prove successful. For the non-religious individual a different channel is required, and this is often found in someone, something or a power outside that person (King *et al*, 1994). Religious belief may not always help the dying person. Faith can be severely shaken at times of crisis and questions such as 'how can God let me suffer like this?' are sometimes prevalent, as is the fear of judgement. Stoll (1989) suggests that people may seek sources of strength, a higher power or being for their spiritual needs.

An understanding of the essence of spiritual care has proved difficult as shown in studies cited by Walter (1994). Nurses were found to call in the clergy as a way of dealing with the spiritual needs of their patients. This is disturbing considering that studies by Harrison and Waugh were published in 1992 long after nursing had claimed a break-through in this area. In view of this, perhaps we need to remind ourselves of the fundamental issues involved with spiritual care.

There are aspects of spirituality, such as genetic make up, temperament, ethnicity, sexuality that are inherent within a person, and this is what makes you, you. On the other hand, there are other aspects that are acquired, such as experience, education, profession, family and even the society in which you are brought up, and this makes you what you wish to be or end up being, (see *Figure 6.1*).

Therefore different people will have variations in the aspects acquired and their sense of purpose may also differ.

However these different people tend to have similar indicators of spiritual health. The following list consists of some of these common indicators:

- humour
- hopefulness
- enthusiasm
- creativity
- sharing with others
- joy
- ability to adapt easily to change
- finding **meaning** in struggle and suffering.

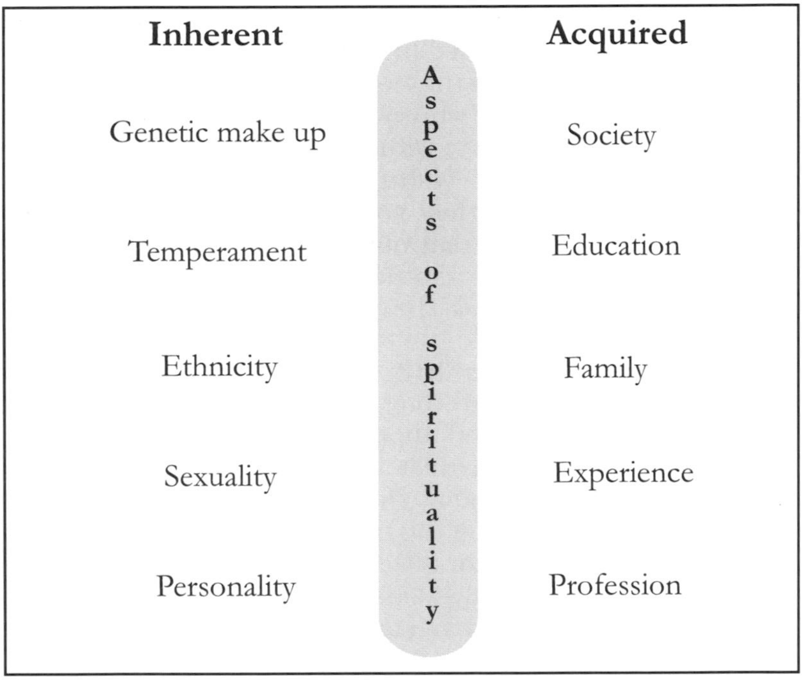

Inherent	Aspects of spirituality	Acquired
Genetic make up		Society
Temperament		Education
Ethnicity		Family
Sexuality		Experience
Personality		Profession

Figure 6.1: Aspects of spirituality

These are only indicators and should be used as such, for example if someone was always creative, but does not seem to be so anymore, one must question the spiritual well-being of that person. The only problem is that healthcare professionals do not always have the knowledge of what this person was like before they became a patient. They often meet them in times of illness, but perhaps speaking to significant others may be a way of gaining this knowledge. Patients who retain all or some of these indicators in their dying may be coping well with their spiritual needs.

It is claimed (Sumner, 1998) that patients may experience two levels of spiritual needs, firstly spiritual distress and secondly spiritual despair. A patient in spiritual distress may show signs of mild anxiety, discouragement, anhedonia, unusual questioning of the role and existence of God or a higher power, expressing feelings of guilt and disturbed sleep. Some may even challenge their own belief and value system.

Spiritual despair is characterised by complete loss of hope, anhedonia leading to refusal to talk to loved ones. The patient may have death wish tendencies often followed by severe depression. At this point patients can refuse to participate in their own treatment regimen. Spiritual despair is the extreme, which should be avoided if healthcare professionals can address the patients needs while in the spiritual 'distress phase'.

There is the argument that people in spiritual distress will benefit from, among other interventions, unconditional love and a non-judgmental approach (Narayanasamy, 1991). A non-judgmental approach assumes that the carer is completely self-aware, and this demands certain under-standing by the carer of his/her feelings and behaviour. Self-awareness has two parts that need understanding before any claim to being fully self-aware can be made. Each individual has an inner as well as an outer self, and most often will be aware of his inner self in terms of feelings, biases, stereotypes, thoughts, beliefs and prejudices (see *Figure 6.2*). However, he may not always be aware of his outer self, which others see through his behaviour, but have to rely on feedback from others. It is important to emphasise that other people will not be aware of inner feelings, but can only make an interpretation through the observable behaviour. For complete self-awareness the individual will need to receive honest feedback on behaviour in order to reconcile it with the inner self. Once this is achieved it is possible that movement towards a non-judgmental approach is achieved. The emphasis on honesty is made intentionally as it often creates conflict in any polite society such as ours, because we tend to say what we believe others want to hear and obviously cause no harm.

A simple example is when I was living in the nurses' home during my training period and one of the student nurses came into the sitting room wearing her new dress. She asked how she looked as we were all going out to a party. What was really obvious to us was that the dress did not suit her and secondly she was far too overdressed for this party. However no one was honest enough to say this, instead we all commented that she looked wonderful. There are so many arguments about this scenario but the fact is we did not honestly offer our subjective judgements, which I believe our colleague student was seeking. Some people would argue that it was kinder this way rather than upset someone who had spent a lot of money on this dress. If this was to be accepted as protecting others then complete self-awareness can never be achieved when it comes to adopting a non-judgmental approach. The dress issue could be seen as trivial but this behaviour tends to occur even with more serious issues. There are similarities between this notion of self-awareness and that of the Johari Window.

Spiritual care is about helping the patient to find inner peace, meaning in illness and acknowledgement of pain, often expressed through questions (but not really questions) of 'why me?' Such questions do not necessarily need to be answered by the carer, but to be viewed as indicators of the patient's need to talk about

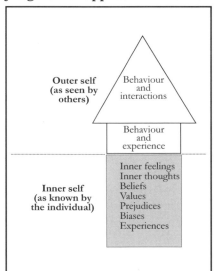

Figure 6.2: The notion of self-awareness

the impending death. The meaning in question here is what Frankl (1984) sees as the primary motivation in life and not a 'secondary rationalisation'. The meaning is unique and specific to the patient in that it must and can be fulfilled by him alone.

The social dimension of care

Social care recognises that the changes due to life threatening illness forces different individuals to review their roles. For the dying person it means not being able to perform his or her role anymore. This may cause immobilisation as shock overwhelms the individual. The dying person realises that there is a mismatch between high expectations or ambitions and the reality of his or her situation. Some people tend to deny this change and may find themselves temporarily retreating. While this is happening to the dying person, the same process may be taking place with close relatives. All these reactions are aimed at achieving some kind of equilibrium within the individual, so that proper functioning is resumed as soon as possible. This is where healthcare professionals can play a leading role in facilitating the achievement of this equilibrium. What we need to bear in mind is that what seems so logical and straightforward for us may not be that simple for the dying person and his relatives (family unit). Their life is filled with 'chaos' and uncertainty which may easily lead to conflict, in either a positive or negative way. Understanding of these positive and negative forces may be central to healthcare professionals in helping the family unit. The whole picture of the family unit needs to be understood in terms of what gaps or roles will be created by the dying person, and who is likely to fill those gaps. Kurt Lewin talks about analysing the forces involved with any change (Lewin, 1951). Some forces are for the change, ie. driving forces, while others are against the change, ie. resistant forces. Before we offer social care it may be worth considering these forces for each family unit. Doing it this way means that we can identify as many negative forces as possible and then prepare ourselves as to how these may be turned into positive forces. It also shows us, the carers, at a glance, which forces outweigh others and therefore where to concentrate our energies. Once these forces have been identified, they should be ranked as the most positive and the most negative. Ranking can be done from one to ten. The following case study highlights how these forces can be identified and ranked.

A family tree is used to understand the family unit (Nyatanga, 1993) based on the family unit of Sid and Joan (see *Figure 6.3*).

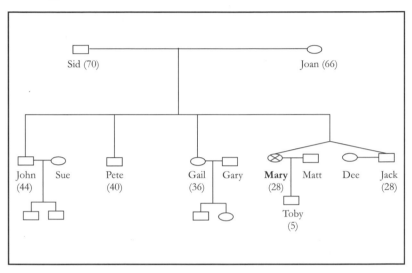

Figure 6.3: Family tree

Case study, background history

Sid and Joan are both retired in their late sixties. They have five adult children, ranging from the age of forty-four to twenty-eight; the youngest of whom are twins, Mary and Jack. John, the oldest son is married to Sue with two boys. Pete has no partner and at forty continues to live at home with his parents. He cares for them both, particularly for his father who, at seventy, is becoming very frail. Gail, the oldest daughter is married to Gary and have two children; a boy and a girl.

Mary and Jack are non-identical twins. Jack has a partner, Dee. Mary is terminally ill with breast cancer and has a partner, Matt, whom she plans to marry in six months time. They have a five-year-old son Toby. Mary's prognosis is poor, being estimated by doctors at less than three months survival

The family is geographically scattered and they have not been emotionally close, with the exception of the twins, Mary and Jack, who are inseparable and live near to one another. Mary is unaware of the seriousness of her illness and she is making plans for her wedding followed by a honeymoon abroad. Jack suspects Mary's illness may be more serious than they had all thought and seeks advice from brother Pete who spoke to the consultant when he drove Mary for her last appointment. Pete thinks it best not to tell their parents due to Sid's poor health. Jack is not so sure that he agrees with Pete's decision and would like to talk to his mother with whom he shares most things. Neither Gail nor John and their families live nearby so they have not yet been told. However, Gail and her husband Gary plan to visit their parents soon to tell them of their plans to emigrate to Australia where Gary has been offered a better job, and is due to start in three months' time.

From the above case study can you identify the positive and negative forces, working for and against the effective family social dynamics as they come to terms with Mary's illness. Can you also rank in order these forces between 1 and 10, with 1 being the weakest and 10 the strongest force. What could be the effects of Mary's illness on the various members of her family? When you have finished you could compare your analysis with the one in *Figure 6.4* done by a colleague, Celia Robinson. If you feel doing this may provoke memories in your own personal life, perhaps you can try and analyse the forces involved in moving house.

This type of analysis is not different from other types of assessment to elicit patient needs. There is obviously going to be an element of subjectivity within a well intended objective analysis using such tools, therefore differences are expected. For example, Pete's care of Sid can also be negative if you felt that he was overprotecting his father to the extent of denying him the right to information about his daughter.

Figure 6.4 shows that negative forces outweigh positive forces. The interpretation may be that a lot more work is required in order to overcome the negative forces or turn them into positive ones. Pete carries the brunt of his parents' care. As healthcare professionals, we must ask certain questions in order to obtain a clearer picture of the situation. For example, how serious is the disagreement between Pete and Jack? Is it feasible for them to form an alliance in telling the rest of the family and help them to come to terms with the situation. Could Mary's wedding be brought forward? Could the emigration plans be delayed and, if so, would that result in Gary losing his new job? Might he then live to regret it or maybe blame it on the illness?

Rank	Positive forces (+ve)	Negative forces (-ve)	Rank
10	Closeness of the twins Mary and Jack	Lack of emotional closeness of other family members	10
10	Pete's presence at home	Sid's frailty	10
10	Pete's support of his parents	Poor health of the parents	7
10	Pete's care of Sid	Mary unaware of her prognosis	10
8	Mary's impending marriage	Most of family members unaware of Mary's poor prognosis	10
		Disagreement of Jack and Pete about telling Sid and Joan of Mary's prognosis	7
		Emigration plans of Gail and Gary	6
		Preparing and helping Mary's partner and son	10
		John keeps himself at a distance to the family situation	8

Figure 6.4: Analysing the forces created by Mary's illness

Once a clearer picture is obtained, specific intervention by healthcare professionals may be needed to draw the family together and facilitate open discussion. Pete may need additional support in caring for his parents; Mary, her partner Matt and son Toby; and possibly Jack may need special help to come to terms with this situation. The healthcare professionals also need to concern themselves with how the news of Mary's illness may be received by Sid and Joan. The range of emotions being experienced here may affect the existing family dynamics. It is possible that the end result may be an emotionally closer family or a widening of the present distance.

Physical dimension of dying

The way a patient and the healthcare professional view the 'dying body' is often the same. However, there may be some differences in perception if the same body was in a lot of pain or discomfort, and the patient, at that time, viewed it as a painful immediacy while the healthcare professional viewed the same body as an object to be examined or, at the very extreme, as a problem to be solved. This apparent discrepancy has a degrading effect on the patient and can often cause conflict. The way forward would be for the healthcare professionals to share the patient's view about his or her body, and together find a way of intervening.

It is well documented that physical ailments often have a bearing on the psycho-social dimensions of the patient. Healthcare professionals need to be aware of this causal relationship so that any care provision is as accurate and effective as possible. Some of the most notorious physical complaints of the dying patient include pain, nausea and vomiting, shortness of breath, constipation, noisy breathing due to excessive secretions, fatigue, dry mouth and pressure sores.

Pain

When a patient is in pain it is difficult to concentrate on anything else. Pain can mean different things, for example, persistent pain may mean one is incurable or going to die (Twycross, 1997). Such physical pain can often have a bearing on the psychological well-being of a patient; the rule is to consider pain in terms of its totality. This means being aware of the concept of total pain (see *Figure 6.5, p.116*) and also realising that such pain is intertwined and may prove difficult to pinpoint or separate. It is now well documented (Twycross, *op cit*) that a patient can experience more than one type of pain at the same time, in which case, a comprehensive and multidimensional intervention is called for. This also requires the use of both orthodox and complementary approaches to control the pain. In palliative circles the rule is to control pain first and then manage it. Pain control is achieved by titrating a quick acting analgesia against the pain. This requires continuous monitoring and adjusting of the analgesia according to pain levels until the pain is well controlled. At this point, pain management should start.

Pain management ensures that patients are pain-free all the time as opposed to waiting for pain breakthrough and then offering them pain relief. Admittedly, some patients may wish to experience some of their pain for various reasons. For example, it is possible for patients to attach meaning to their life through the amount of pain they suffer. For some patients experiencing their pain helps to internalise the reality of their terminal illness. The point to emphasise is that pain management aims to make the patient's pain bearable, ie. something they can live with.

However, if the pain is subsiding for whatever reason, there is also a need to taper the opioid analgesia. There is not yet an agreed formula for doing this, but examining the different schools of thought in specialist palliative care, the general rule is to be more cautious. Opioid tapering can safely be achieved by a 25–35% reduction every other day, while still monitoring the patient for any reactions. Some specialists would advocate a 50% reduction every three days. In this case it makes tremendous sense to use the rescue medication while tapering, and the amount given over 24-hours could guide the next dose reduction. All this forms part of the pain management process on top of talking to the patient about his pain. It is nonsensical to administer small but frequent doses of morphine, because this does not help the patient's pain only the prescriber's own fear of morphine. Such mythical ignorance should be laid to rest once and for all. Each prescriber, particularly those not working in palliative care settings, should liaise with more experienced nurses and doctors in palliative care for guidance. I have always had difficulty in understanding those people who know it all and will not consult others. While this practice may be trying to 'stamp' one's authority on prescribing, it fails to help the pain being suffered by the patient. It is important for all prescribers to think of the patient first because, ultimately, it is the patient who suffers from our mismanagement of the pain.

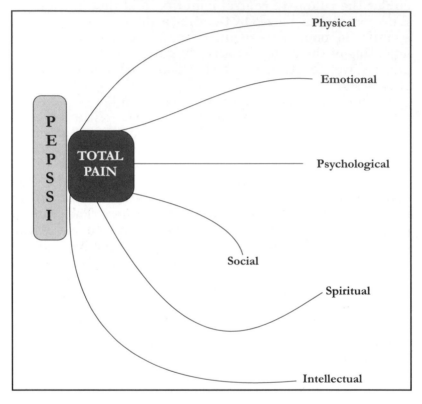

Figure 6.5: The PEPSSI approach to care

Nausea and vomiting

Patients may feel nauseous for several reasons, some of which are iatrogenic in nature, for example, treatment regimes such as chemotherapy. Such iatrogenesis is unfortunate because the treatment itself is intended to palliate distressing symptoms, yet the side-effects end up being equally distressing if not worse.

There may be other causes such as constipation, which

can be alleviated by good bowel care approaches followed by bowel management.

Constipation

This symptom can be caused by opioid therapy, in particular morphine . According to Claud and Tempest (1998) clinicians should understand that the actual need to treat constipation is in itself an indication of failure to prevent it. Constipation should be treated by regular use of laxatives (Lee, 1995) and the laxatives should be titrated until faeces are comfortably soft (Claud and Tempest, 1998). The presence of diarrhoea needs investigation as this could be an overflow from the underlying constipation.

Dry mouth

This is one of the most uncomfortable symptoms which often causes difficulty when speaking, as the lips get stuck to the teeth. The use of mouth swabs, frequent sips of cold water and applying vaseline (petroleum jelly) to lips are some of the local measures that will provide some comfort. Pineapple chunks can be useful for stimulating saliva production, therefore lubricating the mouth naturally.

Claud and Tempest (1998) and Twycross (1997) provide further detailed reading on the above symptoms and other distressing symptoms.

The final phase of illness

The person entering the final phase of an illness will often draw from a kaleidoscopic set of experiences, making that person unique. Each death must reflect this uniqueness in its process. The process should be accompanied by a host of realities that make sense for that person. This is not always easy to achieve but it is important that it is afforded the dying person, because life at this stage is one of ever changing identities from the disease and interactions with others. According to Bertman (1991) the dying person ends up facing a whole range of issues including the following:

* A triangle of interactions between patient and healthcare professionals and patient and family members.

* The loss of control and independence which often leads to helplessness and hopelessness. This also leads to feelings of worthlessness and low self-esteem.

* The dying process may leave the patient feeling psychologically isolated, lonely, vulnerable, alienated and mutilated.

* The spiritual concerns are brought into sharper focus by scrutinising one's relationship with higher powers and/or God (Nyatanga, 1997; Woof and Nyatanga, 1998). It is here that the dying person examines existential issues, including those of the meaning of life and their sense of purpose in the remaining life.

Thinking and doing all these things does not leave the dying person at liberty to die, but tends to add pressure on him and his relatives to ensure that everything is thought about and thought through properly, hence dying becomes so difficult.

According to Lerner (1978) caring for the dying person, although quite arduous can be a rewarding encounter. To the dying person the intervention by the healthcare professionals can be perceived as a real blessing at such a vulnerable time.

Concluding thoughts

Understanding the dying person will ensure that death is as peaceful and dignified as possible. The ideal would be to ensure that the harmonious existence of all the holistic dimensions during healthy living, is also attained during the dying process. In essence, what we are trying to do as healthcare professionals is to help the dying person through their final passage to death. According to Samarel (1995), dying people need assistance and this is often apparent in both the verbalisations and non-verbal gestures. The kind of assistance does not always sit comfortably with healthcare professionals, particularly in the United Kingdom. This assistance should not be misconstrued as mercy killing, but rather it is assisting through the carer's presence and sensitive support. The dying person should be helped so that there is a sense of peace even in the presence of physical discomfort. Any discomfort should be minimised and help given in order to put his/her psychological house in order. Healthcare professionals may need to examine their own 'relationship' with death or, as Samarel puts it, 'reconcile death in themselves'. To be able to help someone achieve peace, you should be able to have peace in yourself first. This may mean accepting death without fear, which has always troubled the human imagination. Fear, if present in the carer, can easily be transmitted to the patient.

Relatives and friends, collectively referred to as the family unit, should be cared for during dying and after the death of their loved one. The healthcare professionals have a duty to inform them of what may be happening with the dying person and the process. The family unit needs to know that the dying person will often need to have some time alone in order to disengage from this life. However, as said before, caution must be exercised so that the dying person does not feel abandoned.

To reiterate, healthcare professionals need to come to terms with their own death first before attempting to help others. Once this is achieved, it becomes quite possible to view patients as living with their dying and not just dying.

References

Bertman SC (1991) *Facing Death. Images, Insights and Interventions*. Hemisphere Publishing Corporation, New York

Burnard P (1998) The last two taboos in community nursing. *J Community Nurs* **12**(4): 4–5

Claud R, Tempest S (1998) *A Guide to Symptom Relief in Advanced Disease*. 4th edn. Hochland & Hochland Ltd, Cheshire

Harrison J, Burnard P (1993) *Spirituality and Nursing Practice*. Avebury, Aldershot

Frankl VE (1984) *Man's Search for Meaning*. Simon & Schuster, New York

Grey R (1996) The psychospiritual care matrix: A new paradigm
for hospice care giving. *Am Journal Hospice & Palliat Care*
July/August: 19–25

King M, Speck P, Thomas A (1994) Spiritual and religious beliefs
in acute illness — is this a feasible area of study? *Soc Sci Med*
38: 631–636

Lee E (1995) *A Good Death*. Rosendale Press, London

Lerner G (1978) A death of one's own. In: Bertman SC (ed)
Facing Death. Images, Insights and Interventions.
Hemisphere Publishing Corporation, New York

Lunn L (1993) Spiritual concerns in palliative care. In: Saunders
C, Sykes N (eds) *The Management of Terminal Malignant
Disease*. Edward Arnold, London

Narayanasamy B (1991) *Spiritual Care, A resource guide*. Quay
Books, Mark Allen Publishing Ltd, Salisbury, Wiltshire

Nyatanga B (1993) Working with emotional pain in palliative
care. *Palliat Care Today II*(III)

Nyatanga B (1997) Cultural Issues in Palliative Care. *Int J
Palliat Nurs* **3**(4): 203–208

Samarel N (1995) The Dying Process. In: Wass H, Neimeyer RA
(eds) *Dying; Facing the facts*. Taylor & Francis, Washington

Sheldon F (1997) *Psychosocial Palliative Care. Good practice in
the care of the dying and bereaved*. Stanley Thornes
(Publishers) Ltd, Cheltenham

Smith R (1986) Toward a secular humanistic psychology. *J
Humanistic Psych* **26**(1): 7–26

Stoll R (1989) The Essence of Spirituality. In: Carson VB (ed)
Spiritual Dimensions of Nursing Practice. Saunders,
Philadelphia, WB

Sumner CH (1998) Recognizing and responding to spiritual
distress. *Am J Nurs* **98**(1): 26–31

Twycross R (1997) *Symptom Management in Advanced Cancer*.
2nd edn. Radcliffe Medical Press, Oxon

Walter T (1994) *The Revival of Death*. Routledge, London

Woof R, Nyatanga B (1998) Adapting to Death, Dying and
Bereavement. In: Faul C, Carter Y, Woof R (eds) *Handbook of
Palliative Care*. Blackwell Science, Oxford

7

Cultural issues in death and dying

Brian Nyatanga

Introduction

The understanding of different cultural needs is important when caring for dying patients. An individual's cultural background influences their behaviour and view of the world they live in. In Britain today 5.5% of the population is of minority cultural groups. This chapter argues that cultures in a plural society like Britain are not static but continually changing. The nature of this change is discussed by looking at the processes of enculturation and acculturation. It is also argued that although some cultural change may take place, some basic rituals at death and dying remain unaffected. This then raises the need for healthcare professionals to be aware of the original (purist) value and belief system of each individual patient's culture, that is before acculturation, and hold that as a broad framework while assessing the current values and beliefs of that individual patient.

The difference between culture and religion is briefly discussed, before selecting a few cultural groups to discuss their beliefs and practices during dying and at death. This is important because the basic tenet of palliative care (which is largely caring for dying people) is to view and treat the patient holistically and if we are to meet the needs of all our patients, then we need to appreciate their varying cultural backgrounds; to understand their expectations during death and dying and how they grieve.

This chapter raises awareness about the different cultures in our society and so appreciates the challenges facing all healthcare professionals.

Before examining the specific cultural issues in death and dying it is important to consider the nature of the cultural changes in today's society.

When providing palliative care to any patient, it is very important that the carer has an idea of the patient's value and belief system. This is even more important in today's Britain which has over the years shifted from being mainly Christian to becoming a more plural society. This shift is also true of other societies around the world. In Britain, the National Council for Hospice and Specialist Care Services (NCHPCS) has indeed recognised the importance of understanding the cultural backgrounds of patients in terms of health. The council (1995) has now published a report on the need for greater involvement by members of the ethnic minorities in palliative care. The council calls for measures that would improve access to hospices and specialist palliative care services by all minority cultural groups to be put into practice. While this may seem an encouraging report, it places enormous demands on all healthcare professionals and other agencies, particularly those in palliative care, to have an increased understanding of the needs of these different cultural groups during death and dying. Also, there are differences within the same group of people, for example, the English will have sub-cultures within them as do Muslims and Jews.

Throughout this chapter information is given which can be readily used in your clinical settings. It focuses on the different cultural beliefs found in the country, highlighting their needs and rituals during dying and at death. This is important as death rituals and funeral rites are the final stage of reconstituting the bond between the deceased and the bereaved. It is not possible to cover every culture in depth, but an overview of the beliefs and care of the dying and bereavement will be provided.

The nature of the changing cultures

The dynamic nature of cultural change is a global phenomenon. Culture is defined by DeVito (1992) as; a relatively specialised life-style of a group of people, consisting of their values, beliefs, artefacts, ways of behaviour and communication. This is a sociological definition suggesting that our life is strongly affected and influenced by our culture. Our cultural background influences the way we view the world and how to behave in it in relation to other people. Any group of people living together tend to produce their own language, laws and mode of thinking as a distinguishing feature from others.

From the above definition, it is implied that culture is transmitted from one generation to the next — a process known as **enculturation**. In other words, culture is something that is learnt and not inherited. For example, a Roman Catholic Bishop is not born celibate, but learns from the teaching of the church and then takes the vow of chastity which subsequently influences his life. Children learn their values from parents, society, peer groups, at school and other similar institutions. When you look at today's Britain with a multitude of cultures, it is evident that the original process of enculturation will inevitably undergo constant change through interacting with other minor or smaller cultures. In any society, the original culture of any group will be influenced and changed according to its exposure to the media, schools, institutions, communities and even direct contacts. The result is often a modification in the original culture, either for survival or because they now share, to some extent, the values and beliefs offered by the other influence. This process is known as **acculturation** (DeVito, 1992) and can be witnessed when the smaller cultural groups, such as immigrant ethnic minorities, modify their culture in line with the host culture. The host culture also changes (although to a lesser extent) as it understands the minority cultures within it.

If, as healthcare professionals, we accept that acculturation exists in any plural society, we cannot afford to hold stereotyped views about any given culture. To do so would make us rigid and unrealistic, denying people's individuality and, as a result, increase the assumptions about the cultural group(s) in question. To assume as Twycross (1994) puts it in terms of pain control, is to make '*An ASS of U and ME* ' (ASSUME).

In a plural society, the original (purist) cultural forms are regularly challenged and someone's impending death will bring these philosophical questions into sharper focus for the individual. Perhaps what we ought to do is hold a framework of each cultural group and how they would behave in their original (purist) form, that is before acculturation, and then assess each individual patient to determine their present value/belief system. It is on the above premise that the information contained in this chapter is based and should be treated.

Some cultures will be resistant to change and therefore defend traditional practices, resulting in inter-cultural conflict. For example, an immigrant family may not modify their values and beliefs even after years of exposure to the host culture. It has been claimed (DeVito, 1992) that open-minded, young people tend to be acculturated more easily than the older generation. It has been suggested (O'Neill, 1995) that even after considerable acculturation, most cultures still retain their rituals and practices at birth, marriage and during death and dying.

Culture *vs* religion

In some cases, culture and religion may have strong associations, but are two different entities. It is possible to find peoples' lives being influenced by both their culture and religion (faith). It is also true to say that some peoples' religion (faith) forms the basis of their life, becoming a way of life, often referred to as a paradigm. For example, if there was a need to change the basis of their life, the change itself can often be seen as a paradigm shift. From their religion, they derive strength and inspiration in difficult times, as can be seen by the comment, 'My strong faith helped me through my problems'.

On the other hand, atheists (people who do not believe in a god) or agnostics (those who believe in silence on the topic god because it is such an abstract concept) still have a culture and spiritual needs that influence their life. As stated above, culture includes values and a belief system. In view of these differences, what may be plausible is to ensure genuine intercultural and religious communication. This should enable people of different values, beliefs and ways of behaving to work collectively for the common goal, in this case, the dying patient.

If we are to understand the needs of the patient and family, then it is also imperative that we start by understanding ourselves and how our preconceived ideas and beliefs may prejudice our perceptions of other cultures. This forms the basis of palliative care philosophy and the provision of culturally sensitive services (Sheldon, 1995). Within the palliative care philosophy are the principles of acceptance and of believing the patient, unconditionally, who may have practices unlike our own. The focus of care shifts from curative to predominantly caring. Caring is about improving the quality of life by blending our competence (skills) with compassion. Maintaining this blend is important in today's healthcare provision where resources are depleted, thereby threatening to erode the fundamental core of caring for the dying patient and family.

The following information is from a selection of different cultures and focuses on the traditional beliefs and care of the dying and bereaved. For more detailed accounts see Rees (1997) and Neuberger (1994) as well as other books listed at the end.

Judaism (Jewish)

Main beliefs

As far back as the 6th century BC the members of the tribe of Judah have been known as Jews. Jews believe in only one God who they believe created the universe (Green, 1993). They place a very high value on the family and also observe the ten commandments of the old testament of the Bible. This makes them practise charity and tolerance towards other people. Although they all believe in the Jewish Holy Book, the Torah, which is made up of the first five books of the old testament, there is now a wide diversity of religious practices among the Jewish community.

Care of the dying and bereaved

According to Neuberger (1999) the Jews would do anything in their power to preserve life, since they believe it to be a special gift from God. They expect the same conviction from the healthcare professionals (HCP) and doctors in particular, as they are believed to be God-sent. Being God-sent, the doctor is expected to have healing powers and should never say the end is imminent (Neuberger, 1994). In view of the way Jews see the doctor as having God's power to heal, there is a potential conflict of expectations as the doctor should not see him/herself as having these powers; placing medicine in a predicament not just with the patient but also with other professionals, ie. nurses.

The Jews would expect the dying patient to continue to eat and drink, which again highlights how difficult it is for them to accept death. Neuberger (1999) sees this behaviour as highlighting the strength of their passion for life. It may be an acceptable aim by most of us in palliative care to achieve a comfortable and dignified death for all the patients we care for, but this concept of a 'good death' is foreign to traditional Jewish thinking. It goes without saying that healthcare professionals need to be sensitive to such issues and establish the patient's prevailing beliefs about their dying.

It is customary for a dying Jew to have psalms recited and they should not be left alone. The Jews believe if you leave a dying person alone he will die more quickly. They are against anyone removing cushions or pillows from under the head, as this will again hasten death. This has implications for healthcare professionals in terms of pressure area care, and other nursing procedures that involve moving the patient. It is here where automatic pressure relieving aides would be satisfactory and culturally acceptable. If the patient has to be moved, eg. in the case of incontinence, clear explanations should be given before the procedure is undertaken.

Once the person has eventually died, the body should be left alone for about ten minutes. A Jewish tradition of placing a feather over the mouth and nose to observe for signs of breathing may be followed. This is a way of ensuring that death has definitely occurred, and before any organs (if needed for donation) can be removed for possible transplants. It is tradition that the eyes of the deceased should be closed by one of their children.

Burial should take place within 24 hours and should only be delayed by the Sabbath (their holy day of prayer and rest). Strictly, Sabbath commences at sunset Friday and ends at sunset Saturday.

A Jewish burial usually involves throwing large quantities of earth onto the coffin using spades in a definitively noisy manner. This is to emphasise the reality of the death to the bereaved and also signals the beginning of bereavement. This is then followed by seven days of mourning (Shiva) with prayers at home every evening. The next phase is 30 days of less mourning (Shloshin) with prayers at the synagogue. After this, there is a period of eleven months rest before the consecration of the tombstone.

It is the Jewish tradition to 'hang on' to life for as long as possible and ritualise death fully as a way of going through bereavement. Care within palliative care should permit Jews to follow their rituals by creating a conducive environment that shows understanding and sensitivity to their needs.

Islam

Main beliefs

Islam means submission to God, and is the religion practised by the Muslims. The Muslims believe in Mecca, their religious centre, and every Muslim has a religious obligation to visit Mecca in Saudi Arabia at some point in their life time. After this visit, Muslim men no longer shave their beard, and they have an outward sign of their maturity. They also wear headgear (a Topi) as a sign of respect. In public, Muslim women cover their heads all the time with a special cloth, as a way of cultural respect.

Muslims believe that they have five duties to perform according to the teaching of Mohammed the Prophet.

- faith (Shahada) declaring their allegiance to god
- prayer five times a day facing Mecca
- giving donations to charity (Zakah). Using the British pound sterling as an example, muslims will donate £2.50 to charity for every £100 savings they have
- fasting for 30 days (Ramadan)
- making a pilgrimage to Mecca (Hajj).

Unlike the Jewish the Muslims believe death to be God's will. Once they realise that they are dying, they may wish to die at home, believing hospitals are irrelevant at this point. They see hospitals as places you go to be cured.

Care of the dying and bereaved

Traditionally a Muslim patient may wish to sit or lie facing Mecca, which is south east. According to leading Muslims, a relative will usually whisper a call to prayer in the patient's ear and then family members will recite prayers round the patient's bed. If no relatives are available, then any practising Muslim can call to prayer and help to give the patient religious comfort.

After death, the body should not be touched by non-Muslims. The head should be turned towards the right shoulder as Muslims believe this will enable the deceased to face Mecca at burial. The body is not traditionally washed nor are the hair and nails cut. The body should be fully covered (from head to toe) by a white sheet. Burial is usually within 24 hours and Muslims do not practice cremation. Muslims believe that the dead person will be asked religious questions about their faith and how they lived their life and that the coffin should be deep enough to allow the dead person to sit up while answering such questions. It is thought that cremation would not allow this important procedure to occur.

Few Muslims believe that their bodies ought to be buried in the country they were born, that is India and Pakistan.

Hinduism

Main beliefs

Hindus believe in different gods and goddesses, who are all manifestations of one god in different forms. They do not believe in a standard way of worship, therefore some may meditate quietly while others go to the temple once or twice a week. Hinduism is the religion of the vast majority of the Indian people. Hindus believe that what an individual does with their life in this world affects what will happen to them in the next world (a belief known as Karma). Hindus are also vegetarians because they do not believe in killing animals for food. The cow is a sacred animal, a symbol of gentleness and unselfish love.

Caring for the dying and bereaved

Most Hindus would prefer to die at home, where they will receive readings and hymns from the Hindu Holy Book (Bhagavat Gita). Some Hindu patients may wish to lie on the floor, a symbol of their closeness to Mother Earth (Rees, 1997: chapter 2). A Hindu priest should be called to perform Holy rites.

After death the family usually wash the body at home. If in hospital and the relatives are not available, the nursing staff can wash the body, but should obtain permission first. Disposable gloves should be worn by staff and the body wrapped in a plain sheet without any religious emblem.

The Hindus prefer jewellery, sacred threads and other religious objects on the body not to be removed.

The priest may tie a thread around the neck and wrist of the dying person as a blessing (Rees, 1997). It is traditional for the priest to sprinkle Holy water from the River Ganges over the dying person's body. The priest may also place a sacred Tulsi leaf in the patients mouth.

Sikhism

Main beliefs

Sikhism was founded by Guru Nanak, who according to Brennand (1992) tried to combine the best of Hinduism and Islam. It was Guru Nanak Dev who first gave women equal rights more than five hundred years ago, but today's society (Sikh) is reluctant to honour these rights. Sikhism originated from the Punjab region in India. The Sikhs believe in one God and it is the responsibility of each Sikh to form their own relationship with God. It follows that each member will have their own way of worshipping. The Sikhs believe in re-birth which will eventually achieve ultimate understanding through a unity with God. They also believe in equality of all people irrespective of colour, caste or creed. The faith of the Sikh is symbolised by five Ks:

- Kesh, uncut hair
- Kangha, wooden comb
- Kara, iron wrist band

- Kirpan, short sword
- Kachha, short trousers.

The Sikhs believe in reading from their holy book — Guru Granth Sahib (Adi Granth), through which they receive spiritual guidance.

Care of the dying and bereaved

A dying Sikh may receive comfort from reciting hymns from the Granth Sahib. If the patient is too ill to recite himself, then relatives or a reader from the Gurdwara (Sikh Temple) can do so instead.

After death the body can be touched by non-Sikhs, but the family may wish to wash the body as part of the rites before laying it out. The five Ks should not be removed from the body, with the hair not trimmed and head covered.

The Sikhs value a calm peaceful expression on the face of the deceased as this will be displayed to those paying their last respects before burial takes place. The body should be covered in a plain sheet with no religious emblem. Sikhs are always cremated, except stillbirths who may be buried.

Buddhism

Main beliefs

Buddhist faith centres on the Buddha who is revered not as God, but a leading example of a way of life. It has been suggested that Buddhism is a paradigm based on the belief that destroying greed and hatred, humans can attain perfect enlightenment. It is believed that greed, hatred and delusion cause suffering to mankind. Traditionally, Buddhists take responsibility for their life and believe that their actions on this earth will be judged in subsequent life. It is therefore important for a Buddhist to behave properly and this includes a strong belief in the sanctity of life. Buddhists condemn abortion and active euthanasia.

Care of the dying and bereaved

Care of the dying will differ among various Buddhist groups but the most important and common consideration is the state of mind at time of death. A Buddhist will want to die with a 'clear mind', free from sedation, as this has an effect on the character of rebirth. This has implications for health-care professionals on the use of drugs that may jeopardise this mental clarity. Clinical experience suggests that most Buddhists are reluctant to take analgesics, especially opioids, as they believe that any sedation is problematic. There is scope in considering 'informational care' that is giving honest information to the patient and the use of complementary therapies, such as acupuncture for pain control.

Buddhists believe that peace and quiet are imperative at death, having a bearing on the character of rebirth. They also need peace and quiet for meditation and some seek counselling from fellow Buddhists. Chanting may be used to influence the calmness of the mind.

When a Buddhist dies it is important that a minister or monk (of the same group) is informed as soon as possible. The usual time between death and burial ranges between three and seven days, dependent on the relevant Buddhist group. Most Buddhists prefer cremation to burial.

Christianity

Main beliefs

The belief in Christianity dates back some 2000 years when Jesus was born in Bethlehem, into a Jewish family. Christianity is the religion of those who are followers of Jesus. It is divided into different groups: the common denominator being the belief in Jesus Christ, the Holy son of God. Christians believe that they can approach God through his son Jesus Christ. According to the teaching of their Holy Book (Bible), Jesus is the result of a virgin birth (a concept that is believed emphatically by some Christians, while others appear more pragmatic about the truth of this theory). Christians believe in Jesus as the Messiah, and a saviour of the universe. Messiah is Greek for Christos, hence the name Jesus Christ.

All Christians believe in an afterlife, either in heaven or hell. This is more of a fundamentalist view and that heaven (often described as paradise, see Luke 23: 43) is the place where those who have followed God's commandments[1] will go and have eternity. Hell is the opposite of heaven where all sinners (those who have not followed God's teachings) would go and be burnt to death. Most Christians, when approaching death, will continually assess themselves and how they feel they have lived their lives on this earth and their chances of a new life after death. It is quite common that those whose faith in God is ailing usually rediscover it as death approaches. This is also true of other cultures and religions. There are cultural differences in the way Christians in different countries view death (Neuberger, 1994a). For example, Christians like Roman Catholics and Protestants in Ireland are much more open than their counterparts in Britain and celebrate death in a way that does not happen in Britain (Neuberger, 19994b). In Britain, death appears to be still viewed as a taboo topic, not because of the pain and loss caused, but perhaps because of fear of the unknown. Death is seen as a source of denial and potential enslavement of the dying and their family. Although attempts have been made by those who believe in 'near death experiences', to explain what happens after death, it still remains the greatest source of fear and uncertainty.

Rastafarianism

Main beliefs

Rastafarians originated from the West Indies, Jamaica and the Dominican Republic in particular. They are descendants of the slave trade families who were forced out of Africa to work in the sugar and other plantations. The Rastafarian movement was first established to strengthen the resistance

---

1 Readers who are not familiar with the commandments are referred to Exodus 20: 1–17 in the old testament of the Holy Bible.

to slavery and emphasis is placed on identifying with mother Africa. A central component of Rastafarian belief is the accession of Ras (Prince) Tafari as the Emperor of Ethiopia in 1930. They believe that the Emperor is a divine human being, the Messiah of the human race who will lead all black people to freedom. Rastafarians respect the old and new testaments as scriptures, but do not consider themselves Christians (Green, 1993). They believe that God's spirit has been reborn in Ras Tafari. Rastafarians believe that they are the true Jews and will eventually be redeemed through repatriation to Africa, their true home and Heaven on earth. Rastafarians do not believe in organised worship and there is no clergy. The belief centres on a deep love of God with the Temple of God being within each individual member's body, which should be kept holy.

Care of the dying and bereaved

Rastafarians are reluctant to undergo any treatment that may contaminate God's Temple (their body) and so western-style treatments may come second to alternative therapies, such as herbalism. Blood transfusion and organ transplants will not be acceptable. Orthodox members of the Rastafarians show their symbol of faith and black pride through their dreadlocks hairstyle, which is not cut at all. After death Rastafarians have a 10-day period of reading the scriptures. Prayers are said in the name of Ras Tafari, the new Messiah.

Paganism

Main beliefs

Paganism is a religious belief centred and maintained orally as opposed to having a Bible (Talmud). Although the Pagans have different practices within paganism, they seem to have some common fundamental principles.

Firstly, it is their belief in a Goddess, which forms the initial focus for their worship. This is the feminine principle. The Goddess has different names, maiden, mother and crone, which when translated represent youth, maturity and death respectively (Prout, 1992).

Secondly, Pagans believe in exercising their capabilities and abilities but without causing harm to anyone. This is the principle of freedom with responsibility. Most Pagans believe in their closeness to nature and are prone to adopting alternative lifestyles.

Thirdly, Pagans believe that they have no control over what happens in their life. This is the principle of destiny. Although this may seem to contradict their second belief, this does not in any way negate their responsibility, but perhaps provides a basis for coming to terms with death and dying.

Finally, they believe in the recycling of their energy after death. This equates with their belief in reincarnation. The recycling of their energy is their way of feeding energy back to Earth. This is usually thought to happen through burial as opposed to cremation.

Caring for the dying and bereaved

Pagans would prefer to die at home where they can prepare positively for death. Pagans have their own spiritual advisors whom they expect to visit even when in hospital. A hospital chaplain would not be acceptable unless specifically requested. A dying Pagan may request privacy to worship with friends and family. In hospitals this request may be made during visiting hours.

Pagans are prepared to donate their organs and receive transplants and transfusions. Following death, according to Prout (1992), last offices may be carried out by nursing staff with no special rituals. Bedside prayers will not be acceptable after death, but can be performed by fellow Pagans just before death. Pagans are in most cases buried and, ideally, they prefer a fellow Pagan to conduct the funeral service.

Readers interested in pursuing cultural issues in palliative care should refer to the following authors: Burja, 1983; Cowles, 1996; Haroon-Iqbal *et al*, 1995 and Jonker, 1996.

Final comment

When all the groups discussed above are being cared for, particularly during death and dying, there are some patients who may not speak or understand the English language. Although healthcare professionals have tried to find interpreters, one concern with the Asian community is using a family member as an interpreter. There are a catalogue of ethical as well as personal dilemmas in such practice. Most Asian people believe that the diagnosis of cancer carries a stigma, therefore the person with a diagnosis would like to maintain his or her own privacy about this. Asking a family member to interpret leaves the patient's secret exposed, denying him his privacy. The patient will often find that his family members become curious about the extent of the illness and the likely prognosis. Most of the family members used as interpreters are the young ones who can speak both languages, and the role often burdens them with emotionally charged information. It is not as if he/she can detach him/herself from the patient afterwards, like healthcare professionals when they go off duty. This young interpreter has to go home with the patient who could be his father, mother or uncle. What happens is that the patient will not go back to the hospital for his next appointment. The family member who is the interpreter feels distressed and is often torn between helping his family and self-protection. One solution might be for the hospitals and hospices to hire the services of professional interpreters who will work alongside specialists in palliative care. This arrangement might also encourage members of the Asian and ethnic minorities to access the palliative care services, or any hospital service.

Palliative care should continue to be sensitive to the unique needs of patients from the ethnic minority communities in order to provide high quality care (Oliviere, 1999).

Concluding thoughts

Throughout this chapter a broad framework has been applied for most cultural groups in Britain today. Within this framework emphasis has been placed on the kaleidoscopic nature of cultures under enculturation and acculturation. What emerges is that cultures within a plural society undergo changes and so it is important to assess each individual's cultural needs while keeping this broad framework in mind. It is vitally important that as carers we should hold principles that value peoples' cultural choices, permitting their beliefs to flourish even when they approach death. This understanding should be demonstrated in the way we assess patients' cultural, spiritual as well as religious needs. More often than not, on admission to our care, agnostics end up giving the Church of England (C/E) as their religion, just because the way we ask questions implies that they should have a religion. Unless we are aware of the cultural differences and adept in our skills of assessing, it is possible that the cultural and spiritual needs of most patients will not be identified accurately. In palliative care, we are looking after the whole person (holistic care) and during the terminal phase, cultural and spiritual needs are often elevated and more prominent.

It is reassuring for any patient to have their care personalised (eg. recognising a birthday). Also, acknowledging the festival of Ramadan to a Muslim confers respect and can have many advantages, including the following:

- demonstrating to the different cultural and religious groups, an understanding of their varying needs, thereby reassuring them and gaining their trust
- raising awareness among carers which increases the access into hospitals and hospices of different cultural (ethnic minority) groups.

This attitude shift may counter the allegations that hospitals, along with other public institutions and their staff, do little to understand the needs of the different cultural groups in this country. This is clearly not the case within palliative care, but if we do not actively show that our care is 'culture deep' we risk being tainted with the same accusations.

It should be the aim of every palliative care setting to provide and guarantee, through various ways '**palliative care for all**'.

Additional information on handling funeral arrangements

Transporting a body for funeral abroad

If after death the family wish to send the body back to its country of origin, certain requirements should be satisfied. Steps must be taken to arrange this although the funeral directors should, in practice, arrange almost everything.

The following should be taken only as a guideline and the fees quoted are likely to differ regionally or to have increased since writing this book in line with other market forces.

The family of the deceased should:

* Contact the funeral director of their choice and inform him of their wish to send the body abroad.
* Register the death (normal procedure) but add that the body is to be transported abroad.
  * instead of issuing the usual certificate of disposal, the registrar will make a copy of the death certificate for the family to give to the funeral director. There is usually a small charge, currently £2.00.

The funeral director should do the following:

* Apply to the coroner for an 'out of England' order, usually granted within a day or two.
* Supply airline carrying the body with 'freedom from infection certificate' which is usually obtained from the doctor who signed the death certificate. The doctor may charge a fee varying from virtually nothing to £15.00. Without this certificate the airline can refuse to carry a body that had suffered from an infectious disease.

* Arrange for a zinc-lined, hermetically sealed coffin (air-tight).
* Obtain a certificate to prove that the body has been embalmed.
* If required obtain a consular seal from the relevant embassy.

Cost

All arrangements can be completed in a matter of days. The cost varies (often by as much as £300.00) since different airlines have different freight charges.

If the body was the subject of a coroner's inquest and the verdict was death by natural causes, there are no problems and the above procedure can be followed. If the death was unnatural, for example murder, drug overdose or poisoning, then the repatriation will not be allowed until the court case is over. In this case, the body will be held in the city mortuary until proceedings are complete. Practitioners need to consider the implications for relatives and especially those who wish to perform rituals as soon as possible after death.

References

Brennand JA (1992) *Funeral Rites in Multi-Racial Society*. Unpublished Research Project. University of Sheffield, Hallamshire, January 11

DeVito J(1992) *The Interpersonal Communication Book*. 6th edn. Harper Collins Publishers, New York

Green J (1993) *Death with Dignity. Meeting the Spiritual needs of patients in a multi-cultural society*. Nursing Times Publication, London

The National Council for Hospice and Specialist Palliative Care Services (1995) *Opening Doors; Improving access to hospital and specialist palliative care services by members of the black and ethnic minority communities*. Occasional Paper 8. NCHSPCS, London: January

Neuberger J (1994) *Caring for Dying People of Different Faiths*. Wolfe, London

Neuberger J (1994a) A Jewish perspective on palliative care. *Palliat Care Today* **111**(111): 32–33
Neuberger J (1994b) Cultural Issues in Palliative Care. In: Doyle, Hawks J, MacDonald (eds) *The Oxford Textbook of Palliative Medicine*. Oxford University Press, Oxford
Neuberger J (1999) Judaism and palliative care. *Eur J Palliat Care* **6**(5): 166–168
Oliviere D (1999) Culture and ethnicity. *Eur J Palliat Care* **6**(2): 53–56
O'Neill A (1995) Cultural issues in palliative care. *Eur J Palliat Care* **2**(3): 127–131
Prout C (1992) Paganism. *Nurs Times* **88**(33): 42–43
Rees D (1997) *Death and Bereavement. The psychological, religious and cultural interfaces*. Whurr Publishers, London
Sheldon F (1995) Will the doors open/ Multicultural issues in palliative care (editorial). *Palliat Med* **9**(2): 89–90
Twycross R (1994) *Introducing Palliative Care*. Radcliffe Medical Press, Oxford

Further reading

Burja J (1983) *Cultural and Social Diversity: A Third World in the Making*. Open University Press, Milton Keynes
Cowles KV (1996) Cultural perspective of grief: an expanded concept analysis. *J Adv Nurs* **23**(2): 287–294
Haroon-Iqbal H, Field D, Parker H *et al* (1995) Palliative care services for ethnic groups in Leicester. *Int J Palliat Nurs* **1**(2): 114–11
Jonker G (1996) The knife's edge: Muslim burial in the dispora. *Mortality* **1**(1): 27–43

8

Funerals: functional or dysfunctional?

Brian Nyatanga

The meaning of funerals

In funereal terms, death becomes a measurement of life, while at the same time, life becomes transparent against the background of death. Death evokes all sorts of reactions and behaviours in us and is a catalyst which, when put into contact with different cultures, precipitates central beliefs and concerns. It can be argued that death is the removal of the most precious thing (life) from this world. This has often attracted comments like timely or untimely, which will also influence how the bereaved express their emotions. Funerals are the most immediate reflective 'vehicle' of remembering the dead. Such remembrance can be either positive, negative or even disruptive. As will be explored in detail later, funerals can be celebratory occasions or, in some cases, sad and painful events.

It may be worthwhile to look at the sociology of death and dying. This will help to put into perspective the role(s) of the funeral. To explore the sociology of death in more detail, the following sources are recommended: Seale, 1998; Clark, 1996; Prior, 1989; Sudnow, 1967.

Death is often compared to the sun (which provides the source of life in the natural order) in that it provides the central force or dynamism underlying life and the structure of the social order. Death is influential in religious circles, philosophies, arts, political ideologies and medical advances. On the other hand, death sells newspapers (depending on who has died and how the death occurred) and may be used as a way of ascertaining the adequacy of social life. Death is used to sell insurance policies, a thriving area of business which has now developed different policies for each type of death, eg. accidental death insurance policy. Death is often used as a basis for comparisons of different cultures and societies on life expectancy, as an indicator of social progress, decline or even stasis.

The role of funerals

One evening my 14-year-old son (during our regular chats) tried to wrestle with the 'what happens after death' notion and why people react in the different ways that they do. He thought that some people feel very angry about someone's death while others celebrate the life of that person. These are obviously ways of coping or dealing with life without that person who is now dead and gone. The anger may be triggered by the fact that death has robbed this person of his life without agreeing or consulting on how and when death should occur.

From an anthropological perspective death has received social recognition through various processes and activities, including funeral rites and rituals. Such ritualistic activities have one common purpose, the disposition of the dead body. One often wonders why most people from whatever culture find it necessary to have some kind of ceremony for this disposition? Would it not be acceptable for a family to dispose of the body quietly without a funeral or any ritualistic practice. But, death should not be seen as an incident affecting the individual and his immediate family (Denison, 1999) as it has a significance for the wider community, who will therefore take part in celebrating the life lived by the deceased and ensure a decent and dignified disposal of the body. The way of disposing of the dead body should adhere to specific contexts and characteristics of the deceased person's value system. For example, a Christian (Roman Catholic) context will be different from an Islamic context of disposing the body. Denison argues that in the Christian context, the words said during disposition are shaped by the theological motivation of that Christian faith, and may not be appreciated by a group with a different faith.

Leming and Dickinson (1998) argue that funerals and their rituals allow individuals to maintain relations with ancestors. It is obvious that not everybody believes in ancestral practices, but funerals still play a part after death. Funerals have the potential to unite family members by physically bringing them together and allowing emotions to be shared, leading to further solidarity. This view is also supported by Bee (1994) who claims that apart from weddings, funerals tend to bring a large gathering of people together, some related and others through friendship or acquaintance.

However, disagreements also emerge particularly over the 'how the funeral should be conducted' aspect (Walter, 1997). This often leaves some family members dissatisfied with the ritual. When a ritual is performed, the intended outcome is to regain control by the immediate family and community over the disruptiveness caused by death. With control comes the repositioning of the bereaved in order to establish new meaning to their life without the deceased.

On a wider scale, funerals are thought to reinforce social status, fostering group cohesiveness and ultimately perpetuating the social structure of a society. Following on from this, there is the argument that society cares for its people in health and illness and through funerals and ritualistic practices, the emotional well-being of the bereaved is promoted. If this is the case then funerals have no benefit for the deceased directly or otherwise, but are there to benefit the bereaved and the community. Bayliss (1996) argues that the bereaved do not gain financially from a death, since funerals are a costly business. Also, they may become an ordeal, even when the deceased was not closely attached to those left behind. Perhaps one example is the national outpouring of grief witnessed after the death of Diana, Princess of Wales. The question Bayliss poses is why we have developed a custom which sometimes causes more distress at an already vulnerable time? This makes dying more difficult, particularly if the dying person is constantly being reminded of the complexity and cost of funerals. Here cost should be viewed, not only in terms of finance, but also emotionally as well as physically.

As there is an increased tendency for the living to organise their own funerals, it would be interesting to explore whether this eases their dying. One positive outcome of this pre-arrangement, might be the benefit to the bereaved in that they do not have to organise the funeral. On the other hand, the pre-arrangement of the funeral might deprive the bereaved of the only immediate therapeutic 'exercise' following the death of their loved one.

Another role played by funerals is put forward by Maloinowski (1984) who claims that funerary rituals play a significant role in opposing or counteracting the centrifugal forces of fear, helplessness and dismay that often follow death. Such rituals help to rebuild the family's weakened solidarity and rejuvenate any shaken morale. This is often achieved through reflection and/or reminiscence.

Such rituals tend to reflect on the good or positive aspects of the deceased's life, while ignoring the negative. For example, I have rarely heard any demeaning accounts at a funeral ceremony, even when it was obvious that during the deceased's lifetime there was hardly anything positive to applaud. Durkein (1954) argues that funeral rituals are intended as a collective expression of sentiment, anything negative would not help the emotional well-being of the bereaved. Another argument put forward by Fulton (1995) is that funeral rituals help to incorporate the deceased into 'the world of the dead' by highlighting all the positive aspects of their life. Going through the actual process of funerals signifies the end of life and the separation of the dead from the living (Fulton, 1995). This may only be temporary and viewed mainly in physical terms as it can be argued that some deceased people tend to continue to maintain some kind of relationship or contact with their bereaved relatives. This will be explored later under the heading 'Living with the Dead' (p.144), but for now the focus moves to how funerals can be different in their functions.

According to Mandelbaum (1959) there are two main types of funeral functions namely; manifest and latent.

Manifest functions are those associated with mortuary rites that are readily apparent, including disposal of the body, helping the bereaved practically and financially, public acknowledgement of the death and demonstration of continued group and family solidarity.

Latent functions are to do with funeral customs, including economic and reciprocal social obligations that are re-enacted at the time of death. They may include restrictions and obligations placed on family members with regard to attire, demeanour, what they eat or drink and social etiquette. Mandelbaum claims that this is important to show family support and togetherness. It is still common practice in most western cultures to wear black at a funeral. Black is seen as synonymous with sadness, a sombre mood and generally that something is not right. For example, black was used to describe the British Government's 'Black Wednesday' under prime minister John Major and chancellor Norman Lamont. The association of black with bad or negative experiences does not help our quest to view death as a natural process of life and to eradicate the taboo of death. A change to a brighter colour might convey a change in mood and perception of death and allow a celebration of life.

It must be pointed out at this stage that funerals and their ritualistic practices are not the invention of the developed homo sapiens or of those in the western world. Fulton (1995) claims that funerals existed well before 3000 BC and it is believed that Ancient Egypt had funerals around the same time.

Living with the dead

It can be argued that the deceased do not really leave us entirely, despite the assertion made above that they enter the world of the dead. The deceased tend to play different and numerous roles in the lives of those still alive. For example, the dead may continue to exercise control over the living by stipulations left in their wills. It is quite common for the dying person to re-write his will from the death bed in hospital, hospice, nursing home and even his own home. While the intention is largely to leave the dying person's house in order, it also adds an extra dimension to consider at a most vulnerable time. Wills often create a point of tension and conflict among the dying person's family, especially if the family members do not receive what they believe to be their legitimate share. This belief is often based on several things, including:

- how close the member was to the deceased
- the caring input given during the illness (usually where the illness is chronic)

- the relationship to the deceased, eg. wife, son, daughter or close friend
- the overall value of the estate of the deceased.

One of the key points to emerge from this is how dying may produce other pressures apart from those emanating from the illness itself, hence dying can be extremely difficult for the dying person and those left behind.

The process of living with the dead can also be seen from the legacy left through their memories, which often take a strong hold on the affairs of the living. Memory is a passion no less powerful or pervasive than love. It prevents the past from fading away. On a non-physical level, the dead person is almost always present with the living. This is because he is too meaningful or precious to the bereaved to be forgotten. One view is that the deceased tend to give the living direction and in some cases a purpose to enjoy life once again. According to Bertman (1979) there is another view which suggests that we need the dead to release us from obligations, open up new potential, give us a sense of belonging and strength to carry on with our lives. Such is the essence of symbolic immortality. Kolakowski (1983) views the memory of the deceased as having an inspirational effect on the living to the extent that they (the living) have made magnificent creations such as the Taj Mahal, the Egyptian pyramids and other monuments. It is plausible to accept and suggest that such memories of the dead help us to bring about continuity and meaning to our existence. This goes a long way to explaining why different governments (despite the different political ideologies) maintain national cemeteries for their fallen soldiers.

Western society also encourages the creation of memorial funds, such as those of Diana, Princess of Wales and recently Stephen Lawrence, the black teenager who was the victim of racist murder in south London. Such memorials serve two main purposes. These are:

- the dead continue to live with the living and not to be forgotten
- lessons are learnt from such a death. In the case of Stephen Lawrence, for example, a better future for all is guaranteed by improving race relations. Lessons can also be learnt from what the dead person stood for and

believed in (eg. Diana, Princess of Wales and her numerous campaigns including banning landmines). Although these deaths may have strong influences on how authorities will act in future in terms of introducing new laws, such laws alone may not be enough to change the hearts or attitudes of all people. Attitudes, as discussed in *Chapter 1* can only be effected, and may take a long time to change or shift.

In some instances statues of particular influential individuals are erected as a way of keeping the dead in 'touch' with the living. However, history confirms that not everyone believes in the immortality of the spirit (Kolakowski 1983), the Russian communists are a perfect example when they decided to embalm the remains of Lenin.

This non-belief in the immortality of the spirit creates another dimension of our relationship with the dead. Memories of the dead can invoke fears in the living. One view is that if the dead are not properly appeased through acceptable rituals then their 'ghost' will create mayhem with the living. The belief in the existence of ghosts was seen by Sir Frazer (1968) as a human belief in the immortality of the soul. This belief is passed down from race to race and generation after generation. What tends to happen is that the living sacrifice their real 'wants' in life in favour of the imaginary 'wants' of the dead. It is from this perception that possible explanations can be ascribed to the different ritualistic behaviours witnessed world-wide. In my home country, I have witnessed some tribes appeasing their dead by pouring home brewed beer over the grave, dancing and ululating all night long. Such a ritual would not sit comfortably with a middle class family in England. Instead, flowers may be the acceptable ritual, although looking back in time, flowers were traditionally used to conceal the smell of the dead body until burial took place. In today's society where there are technological advances to prevent the dead body from smelling, there has been a considerable shift from flowers and some people are opting for money or donations instead.

Remembering the dead through obituaries

One method of remembering the dead found in funerary rituals is the use of obituaries. When obituaries were first introduced at the beginning of the eighteenth century their main aim was to act as funeral notices for the whole community (Leming and Dickinson, 1998), thereby inviting all community people to come and pay their last respects to the dead person. With this historical function in mind, it seems that obituaries have shifted in their aim today. For example, in the United Kingdom, it is not always abundantly clear why or for whom obituaries are written. Proponents of obituaries would argue that they are written for the community to inform them of the death (often viewed in the context of loss) of one of their members. The context of loss here is taken to mean that the community has lost the contribution that the dead person made. It is claimed that obituaries also help to place the bereaved in sharper focus for the whole community to appreciate their grief and, where possible, offer emotional as well as practical support. It is logical to argue that obituaries provide a therapeutic value for the bereaved.

When you read obituaries it becomes obvious that they are not part of everyone's funeral ritual, regardless of culture or other individual differences, but are written for a selected few. When you read obituaries it is plausible to think that those individuals have made personal and significant contributions to society and so are given this rather prestigious biographical summation. In other words, such summations offer a platform for the assessment of the meaning of life by the bereaved and the immediate community. What makes this assertion less persuasive is the fact that not everyone who has made such contributions to society receives a biographical summation of their achievements. Obituaries have revealed that not many women or black and ethnic minorities feature in them, leaving Long (1987) to conclude that obituaries are a characteristic of the middle class white male. Obituaries were also viewed by Gerbner as 'social registers' for the middle class. But perhaps the middle class white male was the one who made the contributions to the community worthy of mentioning. It is therefore only right that their bereaved should benefit from the therapeutic effect that obituaries supposedly provide.

However, history confirms that women and black and ethnic minorities have also made significant contributions to the social order, but receive very little, if any, mention. It is interesting to note that where obituaries for women or ethnic minorities appear, they are almost always relatively shorter than those of the middle class. It is always going to be machtpolitik to argue that the length of the obituary is a reflection of the significance of the contribution to the community by the deceased. It is also not surprising to find that the 'judges' of the value of such contributions emanate from the same middle class background. It is clear that the poor, regardless of their contributions, may not always afford such glamorous summations, therefore the 'poor man's' obituary could be said to be the actual funeral itself and verses printed in local newspapers, often selected from a book.

While obituaries remain narrowly focused on the middle class population, perhaps they could include additional information on how the contributions have actually had an impact on the lives of others. Such information might act as a point of emulation by the present generation while ensuring continuity within the communities. To know that one would leave a legacy of memories to help the living may be one attraction in death.

Funerals: functional or dysfunctional

There are arguments on both sides to suggest that funerals are capable of being both functional and dysfunctional, and this is true across different cultures. Participating in the funeral ceremony of a loved one affords the bereaved a sense of belonging to a larger social community (Mandelbaum, 1959). A funeral offers a platform to express painful emotions in a safe and supportive environment. During a funeral, it is quite acceptable to cry publicly while trying to come to terms with life without the deceased. Many authors including Van Gennep (1961) and Mandelbaum (1959) agree that a funeral is a 'rite of passage' which marks, for the bereaved, the end of life and real separation of the dead from the living. It is from Van Gennep's work that more understanding of the rite of passage is drawn. Van Gennep claims that any ritual that involves passage usually moves from one state to another in a tripartite manner.

This trilogy involves:

1. ***Separation***: the deceased individual is removed from his or her previously held social position or role. For example, the dead person is separated from the living.

2. ***Transition***: the deceased individual is moving between previous social state to a new one and here the individual is excluded physically and also in a symbolic way from society. It is here that the dead is believed to move away from the world of the living.

3. ***Incorporation***: the deceased individual is reintegrated into a new social order. For example, a new social order may be to incorporate the deceased person into the 'world of the dead'. Incorporation is most commonly facilitated by various funeral rituals; we have all probably witnessed or heard of deaths where the body has not been recovered and most relatives will not rest until they have performed their rituals with the body.

Looking at Van Gennep's findings, it may seem persuasive to be simplistic and suggest that in such rituals, there is a beginning, a middle and an end. However the real point to emerge here in terms of funerary rituals is that the middle part (transition) takes centre stage or is focused on during death and bereavement. One speculative assertion would be to believe that funeral rites could help to ease the transition phase for the bereaved, making it imperative to have a funeral. This is a time often characterised by intense emotions, disbelief and a desire to come to terms with what is happening. Littlewood (1993) claims that many researchers believe that there is a real potential in such speculation being accurate, but more work needs to be carried out following Van Gennep's initial thesis.

What may also need researching is whether the length of each transition has any bearing or effect on the overall benefit to the bereaved. In any inquiry of this nature cultural variations should be taken into account.

The other side of this argument is the fact that funerals and their rituals are potentially dysfunctional. There is one argument that suggests that funerals become dysfunctional if they do not change or modify in line with changes of the modern world. The values, whether therapeutic or otherwise, placed upon funerals by our ancestors could not possibly remain static in the face of the changing political and socio-cultural orientations of the modern world.

Funerals can be dsyfunctional if, for example, the cause of death was not natural causes, ie. in the case of death caused by bombing, murder or assassination by another person or a group of people. It is possible and has happened before (Fulton, 1995) that such funerals have caused the death of others through the emotional turmoil created by the first death. It is revenge killing and may cost thousands of pounds in destroyed buildings and other possessions. It is now believed that the after-effects of violent deaths (then relived through funerals) can lead to physical pathological symptoms (Sheatsley and Feldman, 1964) such as headaches, upset stomach and tiredness. There is a tendency to have a preoccupation with the death, feeling dizzy and numb. There is an exception to this in that some murders or assassinations (eg. Dr Martin Luther King) can result in functional funeral rituals, because the mourners try and propagate and bind the philosophy of the deceased, in this case that of non-violence (Fulton, 1995). The funeral then is seen as an opportunity to make a real statement and uphold the philosophy, contrary to expectations of retaliation. Finally, it is important to consider the different levels of our social organisation and acknowledge that one funeral can be functional at one level of social life such as the community, but may not be so at a national level. It is important to argue that every funeral ritual should serve a purpose, but the question that needs to be clarified is, what purpose?

Funeral directing

There is another dimension to funerals in the changing world of business and modernisation. In most developed countries death has become institutionalised. This is witnessed when the disposal of the dead body is done by 'strangers'. The bereaved find themselves paying an undertaker (a stranger to them) to transport and dispose of the body of their loved one. The undertaker and other workers in this line of work are providing a service, which has grown so rapidly that it necessitated a change of name from undertaker to funeral director. The funeral director has an industry, which is charged with a significant function with dead people and their families. This dramaturgical function of handling the deceased's body while caring for the emotions of the relatives creates a need for a director to ensure a fine balance between the business affairs of the organisation and the bereaved peoples' emotions. Rees (1997) claims that the funeral directors and their employees receive professional education and the Association of Funeral Directors set examinations for the employees to take. This can only be a positive way of ensuring that the bereaved are treated professionally and sensitively at a time of distress.

Funeral directing seems to be a thriving business for several reasons, most obviously the increased number of people dying. One other reason is that the funeral director and his service function in communities that are no longer as cohesive and where neighbourhood support is now non-existent. Most families in the developed world are depleted due to working away from home and other demands, and so the funeral director may be the only person available to offer (at a minimal charge) support and comfort to the bereaved. Another possible reason is the death-denying attitude of western societies, with the UK leading the list, which prevents important decisions from being made until death has occurred. The bereaved would not therefore have prepared themselves for the funerary arrangements including 'window shopping' for prices of coffins and other relevant requirements. There are other services which, with close scrutiny, the bereaved may not require, but end up buying them all in a package provided by the funeral director. This sounds as if funeral directors are not regulated, but this is simplistic, because today's public are more knowledgeable, (therefore question more) and the funeral directors will be keen to be seen to be ethical in their practices. Most funeral services perform a remarkable function and there are few pockets of the service which take advantage of those in the throes of grief.

As an example of a caring service, the funeral director arranges (with permission from the bereaved) for the reconstruction of the dead body through embalming, which is arguably the cornerstone of this industry. For the bereaved, embalming makes viewing of the body and paying of last respects a much more 'palatable' experience. This is the time the bereaved are thought to 'store' the last picture and memory of the deceased, with which to live the remainder of their lives.

It is here that perhaps healthcare professionals can play an influential role by providing relevant literature on funeral services as part of the literature given to relatives of a dying patient. It is not uncommon for relatives to ask for details of funeral directors and services from the professional carers. We therefore have a duty to assist the bereaved, particularly at a time when their emotions may cloud their judgement. For the bereaved to make the best possible choice of funeral service, they need information and education. They need information about all the options and prices available. The bereaved need to be assured that it is alright to shop around for the best service and price. The cost of a funeral will vary according to the choice of coffin, whether it's cremation or burial, the number and type of cars required (eg. limousine/hearse) payments for the minister, church and doctor's certificate (if the body is to be cremated) and additional costs for catering if required. The bereaved may also benefit from knowing the different prices for a range of coffins. The choice of coffins is wide and varied and tends to cater for everyone's financial position (see *pages 153–154*).

The information given below shows the general funeral services and the cost implication depending on the type of coffin ordered. The costs are based on current prices in the United Kingdom, which are also subject to change in line with inflation and other factors. The bereaved should be able to compare the cost of the whole package and not just a single item. Some of the services are optional, such as flowers.

Coffin types and prices

Name	*Description*	*Cost*
The Glen	Sapele mahogany effect — white taffeta interior (WTI)	£300.00
The Consort	Gloss teak effect — white tafetta interior	£390.00
The County	Gloss walnut effect with engraved panels — WTI	£455.00
The Herald	Light gloss oak effect with decorative panels single raised panel lid — WTI	£535.00
The Priory	Satin finished oak veneer, antique brass finished handles — white quilted satin interior	£555.00
The Balmoral	Gloss finished oak veneer, moulded panel lid solid wood handles with antiqued brass fittings — white quilted satin interior	£585.00
The Cathedral	Gloss finished mahogany veneer, engraved panels distinctive solid wood handles and pewter finished fittings — white quilted satin interior	£635.00
The Traditional	Solid oak timber, traditional design, double panel raised lid — antique metal handles, embellished satin interior with extra deep fill	£815.00
The Opal	Solid oak construction, high gloss dark oak finish — six antique bronze finished cast metal handles — satin interior	£925.00

There is also a range of high quality caskets constructed in either steel or solid timber and the cost may range from £735.00 for the Sentinel casket to £2,500.00 for the top of the range, the Regent casket.

General information on a funeral service

The average cost of a funeral service is about £1,250. This includes initial consultations, paperwork, and overheads. The cost will increase to £1,550 if two limousines are required.

Transportation: This includes moving the body to the funeral director's premises and placing the final disposition. Provision of a hearse will cost £120.00, and a limousine will be £90.00. Excess mileage, that is over and above 20 miles, will be charged at £1.00 per extra mile.

Care of the body: This includes embalming and dressing the body, £30.00.

Facilities: This includes cost of viewing, and funeral or memorial ceremony if it is held at the funeral premises. Usually there is no charge for viewing the body even outside normal working hours. Use of the chapel for overnight vigil will cost £100.00. There is a surcharge of £100.00 on Saturdays and Sundays for using a funeral director and up to four of the staff.

Optional facilities: This includes flowers, music, obituary notices and if the director pays a third party to do a job, this cost is added on. It is helpful to find out whether there are any other charges, often listed under miscellaneous. Once a fuller picture of the service and cost is obtained the bereaved is in a better position to make a decision.

The use of coffins and caskets will have varying costs, for example, the Regent Casket will cost £2,500.00 and the basic coffin, the Glen, will cost £300.00. While it is important to know about these varying costs, it is more important to ensure that the bereaved is aware that the amount spent on a funeral does not necessarily reflect how much you loved the person who has just died. The key factor is sensibility and affordability.

Concluding thoughts

Throughout this chapter some of the roles and functions of funerals and their rituals have been discussed. The funeral rituals tend to differ according to the cultural background of the bereaved family. However, the funerary practices witnessed in different cultures all serve a similar purpose, to dispose the body of the deceased. The rituals performed signify a variety of things, such as; a celebration of the deceased's life, bidding farewell to the deceased, permission to carry on with life for the bereaved, or setting in motion the transition of the dead to another level of life or existence. Funeral rituals tend to form part of a people's solidarity within a family, community or even society. When viewed from this perspective, funerals are a powerful means of bringing people closer to each other and allowing life to go on after death. This kind of ritual or ceremony is perceived as forming the functional part of funerals. Obviously, there is the other side to this argument: if the funeral ritual fails to serve its intended purpose, the outcome could be seen as dysfunctional.

Funerals and their rituals are seen as the last act of showing respect for the dead and internalising them into the memory of the living. Internalisation allows for synergy of emotional activity to occur (which is contrary to the teachings of Freud), ie. the bereaved carries on with his or her life and can invest in others, while simultaneously investing energy in the deceased person. Internalisation allows the bereaved to choose when to remember their dead and when to get on with their lives. These are real choices at difficult times, and the bereaved would be left guilt-free because they have the opportunity to attend to both the deceased and their own life. This would also ensure a healthier state of mind for the bereaved and a return to some kind of social normality for them. Death should not result in emotional imprisonment for the bereaved. It is important for theorists and practitioners to be more sensitive to human feelings and allow the uniqueness of that individual (particularly when bereaved) to flourish without theoretical entrapments. This point, among others, will be developed in the next chapter where arguments are made to move away from staged theories. There is obviously a great need for us all to **listen** to what the patient/bereaved really want. As professionals we can play our part in making dying, death and bereavement a more personal and less difficult an experience to go through.

References

Appleyard B (1999) Death of a dream. *Sunday Times,* March 7th: 4

Bee H (1994) *Lifespan Development.* Harper Collins Publishers, New York

Bayliss J (1996) *Understanding Loss and Grief.* National Extension College Trust, Cambridge

Bertman SL (1979) *Facing Death. Images, Insights and Interventions.* Hemisphere Publishing Corporation, New York

Clark D (ed) (1996) *The Sociology of Death.* Blackwell Publishers, Oxford

Denison K (1999) The theology and liturgy of funerals: A view from the church of Wales. *Mortality* **4**(1): 63–74

Durkein E (1954) *The Elementary Forms of Religious Life.* Allen & Unwin, London

Frazer JG (1968) *In Man, God, and Immortality: Thoughts on human progress.* Cambridge Trinity College Press, Cambridge

Fulton R (1995) Contemporary funeral practices. In: Raether HC (ed) *Succesful funeral service practice.* Englewood Cliffs, Prentice Hall, New Jersey

Kolakowski L (1983) 'The Mummy's Tomb'. *New Republic* **33**: July 4th, 1983

Leming MR, Dickinson GE (1998) *Understanding Death, Dying and Bereavement.* 4th edn. Harcourt Brace, Philadelphia

Littlewood J (1993) The denial of death and rites of passage in contemporary societies. In: Clark D (ed) *The Sociology of Death.* Blackwell Science, Oxford

Long G (1987) Organisations and identity: Obituaries 1856–1972. *Social Forces* **65**(4): 964–1001

Mandelbaum D (1959) Social uses of funeral rites. In: Feifel H (ed) *The Meaning of Death.* New York, McGraw-Hill

Malinowski B (1984) Death and the reintegration of a group. In: Malinowski B (ed) *Magic, Science and Religion and Other Essays.* Doubleday, New York

Prior L (1989) *The Social Organisation of Death. Medical discourse and social practices in Belfast.* Macmillan, London

Rees D (1997) *Death and Bereavement. The psychological, religious and cultural interfaces.* Whurr Publishers, London: chap 5

Seale C (1998) *Constructing Death. The sociology of dying and bereavement.* Cambridge University Press, Cambridge

Sheatsley PB, Feldman JJ (1964) The assassination of President Kennedy: A preliminary report on public relations and behavior. *Public Opinion Quarterly* **28**: 189–215

Sudnow D (1967) *Passing on: The Social Organisation of Dying.* Englewood Cliffs, Prentice-Hall, New Jersey

Van Gennep A (1961) *The Rites of Passage.* University of Chicago, Chicago

Walter T (1997) *The Revival of Death.* Routledge, London

9

Rethinking loss and grief

Jean Bayliss

This book has presented readers with a range of perspectives on death and dying. The unique experience of dying and bereavement has been viewed through a prism, reflecting and refracting the light of insight from a variety of angles. Throughout the book there is an awareness that however many facets of the prism are explored and however many general principles can be shared and agreed, the experience of dying and death is uniquely individual. As a patient once said to me after having been told by a variety of people (some of them professionals) that he was 'going through the grieving process',

> *Why don't they forget their theories — I am the one who's dying, and it's happening here, not in a book.*

This final chapter, is written from a personal perspective and aims to sum up the views expressed in the book, by focusing on the need to value the theory, but to keep the individual in mind. This approach may be a step toward making dying less difficult for the individual. The personal perspectives have arisen from several sources: counselling practice, clinical supervision, training others in understanding and working with loss and grief, personal experience and a growing concern that the received wisdom about the so-called 'grieving process' did not seem accurately to describe what many grieving people were experiencing. Indeed, it was an angry outburst by a young bereaved father of three which first prompted me to look again at what actually seems to be real for grieving people. He declared:

> *I am **not** in a **process** — this isn't like a can of beans on a conveyor belt! I don't think I'm going anywhere, unless it's round in circles.*

The work of Julie Ann Wambach (1985) has confirmed that there seems to be a fixed belief in a 'grieving process' and my own research suggests that many helpers and counsellors also think that a process exists and that it is, for the most part, linear. Grieving people, it is suggested, go through stages or phases or work through tasks. While these formulations may well be true and helpful for some people to be aware of, my concern is that they may be used prescriptively, rather than descriptively.

The valuable pioneering work of Elizabeth Kübler-Ross (1970) gave us a model of what may happen in grief. Her model of denial, anger, bargaining, depression and acceptance has been consistently used in terminal care training and is sometimes used to describe bereavement grief (George, 1992).

It seems unlikely that someone with the vision and humanity of Kübler-Ross would have expected dying (or bereaved) people to march obligingly through these five stages in order. Yet the model is frequently used very rigidly. Occasionally, too, an aura of disapproval seems to exist around those who 'get stuck' in one or other of the stages, or who (tiresomely?) stay 'in denial'. I have myself supported an oncology nurse who was under considerable pressure because, 'You're not getting them through to acceptance quickly enough'. The concept of 'acceptance' seems itself to have gained mythic proportions of an almost beatific state — which is not how Kübler-Ross herself defined the final stage anyway. The more recent adaptation of the Kübler-Ross model also has a linear feel to it,

- shock
- denial (not disbelief)
- anger
- guilt
- fear
- anxiety
- despair/depression
- acceptance/resignation.

Indeed, while I have seen in a dying person's isolation, envy, bargaining, depression, and acceptance, I do not believe that these are necessarily 'stages' of the dying process, and I am not at all convinced that they are lived through in that order, or, for that matter, in any universal order.

What I do see is complicated clustering of intellectual and affective states, some fleeting, lasting for a moment or a day or a week, set not unexpectedly against the backdrop of that person's total personality, his 'philosophy of life' (Schneidman, 1977).

In a similar fashion, thanatologist Mansell Pattison states:

> *I find no evidence to support specific stages of dying.*
> *Rather, dying patients demonstrate a wide variety*
> *of emotions that ebb and flow throughout our entire*
> *life as we face conflicts and crises. It does seem*
> *misleading, then, to search for and determine*
> *stages of dying.*
> *Rather, I suggest that our task is to determine the*
> *stresses and crises at a specific time, to respond to*
> *the emotions generated by that issue, and, in*
> *essence, to respond to where the patient is at in his*
> *or her living-dying.*
> *We do not make the patient conform to our idealized*
> *concept of dying but respond to the patient's actual*
> *dying experience.*
>
> (Wass *et al*, 1988)

Why is it, I wondered, that helpers adopt these models (sometimes, perhaps, without reference to their original formulations)? Why do we prefer a model, rather than accepting that grieving people are living people, who 'do their own thing'? My thoughts were summed up by Dee Cooper (1991), a research assistant, writing 17 years after the death of her son:

> *I suspect that stage models and frameworks of grief*
> *and words like resolution have more to do with*
> *professionals containing their anxieties than reality.*

It may also be that when confronted with the chaos of experiencing the emotional, cognitive, behavioural and physical dimensions that we call 'grief', we distance ourselves by applying a model, because the model feels safer than the chaos.

Although his model is not especially new, it is interesting that Weisman's model of an appropriate death has not gained the status of the linear models of dying (Weisman, 1984). The model offers carers, whether professionals or not, a challenge to achieve with and for a dying person a death that is appropriate to his or her unique experience. It may be significant that Weisman avoids the term 'good' death, with all the controversy that the term arouses. He suggests that we aim to help a dying person in four areas:

- by reducing conflict
- by enabling a death which is compatible with their views of themselves and their achievements
- by preserving or restoring relationships
- by fulfilling some of the dying person's expressed aims.

In some senses, these may seem like modest aims, but they are active and require a strong commitment to communication. Most of all they require **us** to **engage actively** with the dying person, rather than approaching them with a predetermined set of stages that they may be 'in' and feeling helpless when they are not.

In an attempt to develop a non-linear model, Prunkl and Berry (1989) considered how the dying (or grieving) person may change almost from minute to minute, and handle a variety of stimuli both external and internal in a variety of ways. They offer us their four room model.

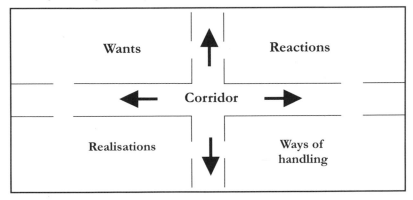

Figure 9.1: The four-roomed model (Punkl and Berry, 1989)

They asked helpers to reflect that if the 'house' is seen three dimensionally, a person may move between each of the 'rooms' almost continually or rest in one for a while. They found no evidence that stages occurred. The different rooms represented changing emotions and situations (for example, 'realisations, wants, reactions and ways of handling') as the person moved and crossed the corridors.

A circular model was suggested to me by a patient of my own who saw his grief as 'swinging about' (see *Figure 9.2*).

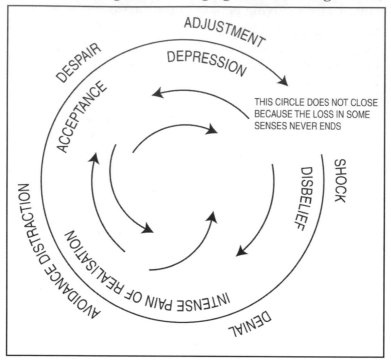

THIS CIRCLE DOES NOT CLOSE BECAUSE THE LOSS IN SOME SENSES NEVER ENDS

Figure 9.2: A circular model of grief

If we are to help people facing the imminent loss of all that is dear to them and the loss of life itself, perhaps we need to examine more closely why we cling to formulations that may well distance us from people and, equally, may not reflect what is actually happening for the person. Perhaps we should 'forget order and work with chaos'.

Terms like 'grief work', and 'working through' have almost become the lingua franca of bereavement and seem to have become separated from their original psychodynamic and psychoanalytical contexts, rather as 'the grieving process' seems to be regarded as fact. The question I found myself asking about the bereaved clients/patients I was trying to help was what exactly is 'grief work' (now that it no longer has Freud's theory attached to it)? Is my client really 'working **through**'? It often seems more as if she/he is working **at**. And 'which process?' Is it tasks, stages, phases; and, if so, how many? It seems to vary from model to model. There has recently been a significant groundswell of thinking which challenges linear or sequential models of grief, while acknowledging that their framework can be helpful to some people sometimes. The concern is that a too rigid adherence to any model can mean that a grieving person who does not, obligingly, go through 'the process' may be seen as 'abnormal'. There is anxiety that grief, the natural reaction to loss, can in this way be pathologised. The sequential models which have, perhaps, had most influence on bereavement counselling/therapy are those of Worden (1991) and Parkes (1986), both of which come from a psychodynamic root. Worden's 'tasks of grief' model suggests that the bereaved 'work through' a series of tasks to resolve their grief. These tasks were originally:

• to accept the reality of the loss
• to experience the pain of grief
• to adjust to an environment no longer containing the loved one
• to reinvest emotion.

The final task has been adjusted to 'to relocate the lost one' in order to move on with life; Worden's revision seeming to mean that rather than reinvesting the emotions and hopes originally invested in the deceased (a Freudian concept), the bereaved work to find a new place in their emotional lives for the deceased. This model had been offered to the young father I quoted at the start of this chapter, who said, of the first three 'tasks' that 'to have done any of that **in order** would have been a luxury'. Five years after his wife's death he often found himself disbelieving the reality that she was no longer with him, yet he was functioning well and in no sense could be seen as grieving abnormally.

Parkes' model was described by Rubin (1996) as a 'pathway' along which the bereaved 'progess'. This consists of:

• numbness
• searching and yearning
• disorganisation
• reorganisation.

This was used as the initial training model for CRUSE, the UK national bereavement care charity. It may be that the notion of 'progress' is one of the reasons why there are increasing challenges to a sequential view of grief. 'Progress' implies that those who move along the pathway are somehow 'doing well' and, more worryingly, that those who do not grieve in any ordered way are somehow, as one respondent in my own research put it, 'not trying to work through the stages of grief'. There has for some time been a movement away from setting time boundaries for the stages (amazingly in the 1940s, perhaps because of the war, Lindeman [1944] proposed 'recovery' over four to six weeks), but there is still some sense that grief should be time limited if it is 'normal'. This seems to be linked to the necessity of experiencing (or working through) painful feelings in order to 'let go', another common term in the language of bereavement. If the bereaved either do not experience those feelings intensely or if the feelings persist, grief is often labelled as 'abnormal' and may be pathologised (Raphael, 1983: 59–60). The work of Wortman and Silver (1989) is especially challenging of these formulations of bereavement grief. They suggest that there is a contradiction somewhere at the heart of theory. Their research did not find universal evidence of the extreme distress or depression which Bowlby (1980) and others have seen as virtually essential for 'healthy' grieving; nor did they find that those who did not exhibit intense grief reactions were denying it, or 'in denial', but rather the reverse. The contradiction they cite is the popular belief that those who do not experience the pain intensely will, at some later point, suffer problematic reactions. If this were so, those who experience intense pain should logically adapt better to their bereavement. Yet the opposite seems to be true — those most distressed early on (ie. who have experienced the pain of grief, Worden's task two) are more, not less, likely to be depressed later on. They say,

> *The data clearly suggests that 'absent grief' is not necessarily problematic..., delayed grief is far less common than clinical lore would suggest.*

They suggest that there is little empirical evidence that not 'working through' tasks or stages will lead to what one worried client once described as, 'a fear that it will sneak up on me and get me when I don't expect it' because her grief was not going along the recommended route. Wortmann and Silver (1989) also challenge any notion of time limited grief. Parkes and Weiss (1983) themselves were surprised at the ongoing grief of widows, but Wortman and Silver see it as normal and concur with the experience of Dee Cooper, quoted earlier, that grief does not follow a fixed pattern in time or in intensity.

Some interesting work in this respect has come from a study of bereaved people in New Zealand. The findings of this study by Tonkin (1996) can be represented graphically (*Figure 9.3: A,B,C*). Soon after the bereavement the grieving person felt 'all loss' (see *Figure 9.3: A*), and it was predicted that over time the grief would diminish, while the person would remain, as it were, the 'same size' (see Figure *9.3:B*). Yet what happened over time was that the grief stayed the same size, but the person grew round it (see *Figure 9.3: C*).

This confirms the experience of many I have counselled who report a strengthening of themselves, and an increase in their understanding of themselves and of their compassion for others. This is not to say that some grief is not exceptionally complex and complicated, but that to label grief as 'pathological' because it does not conform to models may well be to deny the positive effects it can have.

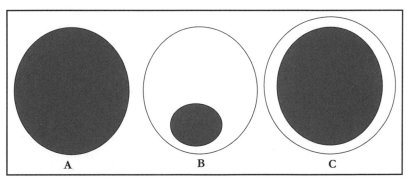

Figure 9.3: Growing around grief (Tonkin, 1996)

The strong influence of Bowlby's attachment theory has also led to some rethinking of bereavement grief. The view that for a healthy adjustment to a bereavement to take place, the bonds of attachment need to be broken has been contested. Tony Walter (1996) concurs with the research carried out by Silverman and Nickman (1996) that far from detaching from the deceased, the bereaved retain very strong attachments, although the relationship and dynamics of the attachment change over time. In *Bereavement and Biography* Walter points out how an event like the funeral can enlarge and extend our understanding of the deceased, changing the nature of the relationship. He also points to the need the bereaved feel to talk about the deceased — in the linear formulations this might be seen as coping with denial or checking the reality of the loss, but Walter sees it more as building the new relationship with the dead. We can, in a sense, all be our own researchers in thinking about how we still relate to those who have had a significant role in our lives. I am well aware of my tendency to 'check out' how my parents might react to or value events in my own life, for instance. Bereaved people frequently say things like, 'He'll always be with me', 'I often just talk to her', 'I look to him/her for advice' and so on, thus their bonds with the deceased are renewed but not in any pathological sense.

Noticing that a desire to stay attached (with no sense that this might be morbid or unhealthy) is the norm in many cultures and was what led, in part, to Margaret Stroebe's imaginative way of looking at grief as non-sequential. From diaries of the bereaved and from practice and observation she noticed that grieving people seem to oscillate between active 'working through', breaking bonds, expressing feelings (loss orientated, as she calls it) and allowing themselves to be distracted, to take on new roles, take up new activities (restorative) (see *Figure 9.4*). Stroebe does not dispute that some aspects of the sequential models may well be real, but that they are not experienced in any kind of order, but more in the way that we deal with any of life's stresses, by sometimes confronting them and sometimes 'putting them on the back burner' as one teenager described his grief to me after the death of his sister.

Finally, it is evident that many of the symptoms of depression are very similar to some of the manifestations of grief. Cognitive-behavioural therapy is one of the few counselling/psychotherapy interventions which offers itself for rigorous evaluation and seems to be particularly

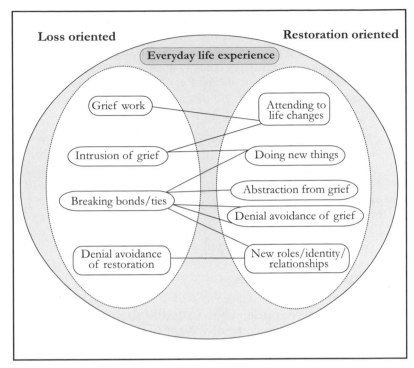

Figure 9.4: A dual process model of coping with grief (Stroebe and Schut, 1995)

successful with clinical and reactive depression. It would seem sensible to use cognitive-behavioural techniques to help grieving people, yet most counselling seems to focus on the affective aspects of grief, urging the grieving person to express or 'work through' a range of powerful feelings. Grief is, of course, very powerful in the feelings it evokes, but it is also experienced cognitively, physically and behaviourally and it may be that as helpers we need to focus on these areas too? To date there is little work in this field but one interesting piece of research suggests that focus on cognitive-behavioural factors could be of great help to grieving people (Power and Wampold, 1994). Grief is, in a sense, the greatest source of stress most of us will experience and perhaps we can learn from techniques of stress management, which are mainly cognitive-behavioural. Power and Wampold attempted the techniques, for example, differentiating devaluing the deceased and attending to life tasks; engaging in health promotion; attributing personal meaning and identifying prominent themes to assist confusion. Their results are very promising and will perhaps encourage more work and research in this largely unexplored (as far as grief is concerned) area.

What conclusions can be drawn from all this challenge? As long ago as 1961 Bowlby said,

> *The painfulness of new ideas and our habitual resistance to them, can also be seen in the (grief) context. The more far reaching a new idea, the more disorganisation of existing theoretical systems has to be tolerated before a new and better synthesis of old and new can be achieved.*

Concluding thoughts

It is a constant reminder that valuable though models may be they are not, or should not, be set in stone: each person's grief is unique to them. This helps me to examine my practice carefully, to be sure that I am not imposing models on anyone or using them as some kind of prescription or panacea, since the only person they would then help is me. Above all, it helps me to listen to this person's pain and not that theorist's model.

Dying and death bring sharply into focus the profound questions, 'Who am I?' 'What makes me, me?' The imminent loss of self, and for the bereaved, the loss of who the deceased was, are among the most disturbing aspects of loss and their very nature means that they are rarely addressed by carers, either professionally or informally. The sense that we cannot answer these questions for ourselves makes us wary of exploring existential or spiritual issues with the dying or bereaved. This apparent deficit is perhaps why we need models as a defence. Maybe we should follow Jung's advice,

> *Learn your theories as well as you can, but put them aside when you touch the miracle of the living soul. Not theories, but your own creative individuality must decide.*

References

Bowlby J (1961) Processes Of Mourning. *Int J Psychoanal* **42**: 317–340

Bowlby J (1980) *Attachment and Loss*. Volume 3. Basic Books, New York

Bowlby J (1981) Psychoanalysis as Natural Science. *Int Rev Psychoanal* **82**

Cooper D (1991) Long-term grief. *Br Med J* **303**

George H (1992) Psychological Support in Death and Dying. *Resurgam*

Jackson EN (1957) *Understanding Grief*. Abingdon Press, Nashville

Jung CG (1953) Jung's Psychology. In: Fordham E (ed) *An Introduction to Jung's Psychology*. Handsworth Pelican, London

Kübler-Ross E (1970) *On Death and Dying*. Tavistock, New York

Lindemann E (1944) The Symptomatology and Management Of Acute Grief. *Am J Psychiatry* **101**

Parkes CM, Weiss RA (1983) *Recovery From Bereavement*. Basic Books, New York

Parkes CM (1986) *Bereavement: Studies of Grief in Adult Life*. Penguin Books, London

Pincus L (1974) *Death and the Family: Management of Acute Grief*. Pantheon Books, New York

Power LE, Wampold BE (1994) Cognitive — behavioural factors in adjustment to adult bereavement. *Death Stud* **181**

Prunkl PR, Berry RL (1989) *Death Week*. Hemisphere Publishing Corporation, New York

Raphael B (1983) *An Anatomy of Bereavement*. Hutchinson, London

Rubin S (1996) *Continuing Bonds*. Taylor and Francis, Philadelphia

Schneidman ES (1977) Aspects of the Dying Process. *Psychiatr Annals* **8**: 25–40

Silverman PR, Nickman SL (1996) *Continuing Bonds*. Taylor and Francis, Philadelphia

Stroebe M (1992) Coping with bereavement: a review of grief. *Omega* **26**: 19–42

Stroebe M, Schut (1995) Helping the bereaved come to terms with loss. In: *Bereavement and Counselling*. Conference Proceedings. St George's Mental Health Sciences, London

Tonkin L (1996) Growing around grief. Another way of looking at grief and recovery. *Bereavement Care,* Cruse, London

Walter TA (1996) A new model for grief, bereavement and biography. *Mortality* **1**: 7–25

Wambach JA (1985) *The Grief Process as a Social Construct.* Omega **16**(3)

Wass H, Neimyer RA (1988) *Dying, Facing the Facts.* Taylor and Francis, Washington

Weisman A (1984) *The Coping Capacity.* Human Sciences, New York

Worden JW (1991) *Grief Counselling and Grief Therapy.* Springer, New York

Wortman CB, Silver RC (1989) The myths of coping with loss. *J Counselling Clin Psychol* **57**(3)

Index

A

abortion 130
acceptance/resignation 159
accountability 57
acculturation 3, 16, 121–124
act-utilitarians 84
adolescence 4
adulthood 8
affective dimension 15
   ~ of an attitude 2
agnostics 5, 124
analgesia 90, 115
analgesics 131
anger 159
anti-cancer treatment 50
anxiety 6, 13, 159
aromatherapy 64
artefacts 122
artificial hydration 64
atheists 5, 124
attachment theory 165
attitude 1
   ~ to death 17
attitude formation 5
attitude orientations
   ~ death denied 8
   ~ death of the other 8
   ~ death of the self 8
   ~ tamed death 8
attitudes
   ~ contemporary
     towards death 7
   ~ crystallisation of 4
   ~ towards death 1
authoritarian organisations 57
autonomy 81, 88–90, 97

awareness levels
   ~ of death 16

B

behavioural dimension 2, 15
beliefs 2, 105, 108, 122, 124
beneficence 31, 81, 90
bereavement grief 165
bowel care 117
Brompton Cocktail 63
buddhism 130
burial 126, 128

C

cancer centres 64
cardiopulmonary
   resuscitation 65
care
   ~ generalisations of
     53
caring 101, 125
childhood experiences 3
children 3
christianity 131
clinical governance 60
closed awareness 19
cognitive dimension 15
   ~ of an attitude 2
cognitive-behavioural
   therapy 166
communication57
   ~ patterns of 19
communication skills 59
complementary approaches
   115
complementary therapies 63